The Medically Based
No-nonsense Beauty Book

THE
MEDICALLY BASED
NO-NONSENSE
BEAUTY BOOK

by Deborah Chase

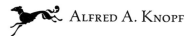 ALFRED A. KNOPF   NEW YORK   1974

THIS IS A BORZOI BOOK
PUBLISHED BY ALFRED A. KNOPF, INC.

Portions of Part I, "The Skin," were previously published in *Family Circle* and *Ms. Magazine.*

Grateful acknowledgment is made to The Metropolitan Museum of Art for permission to reprint three photographs, of the following sculptures:

"Antiquities Egyptian Sculpture Busts XIX dynasty"—Head of a King (probably Rameses, complete statue 1292–1225 B.C.). Rogers Fund, 1934

"The Lady with the Primroses after the marble in the Bargello" attributed to Leonardo da Vinci—1475. Rogers Fund, 1965

"Georgia O'Keeffe Head" by Gaston Lachaise. Reprinted here by permission of Georgia O'Keeffe and The Metropolitan Museum of Art, The Alfred Stieglitz Collection, 1949

The author also wishes to acknowledge the American College of Physicians for permission to reprint two photographs of "Smokers' Wrinkles" from *Annals of Internal Medicine,* December 1971. Copyright © 1971 by the American College of Physicians.

Library of Congress Cataloging in Publication Data:

Chase, Deborah, date.
The medically based no-nonsense beauty book.

1. Beauty, Personal. 2. Women—Health and hygiene.
3. Cosmetics. I. Title. [DNLM: 1. Beauty culture.
2. Skin. QT275 c487m]
RA778.c38 1974   646.7'2   74-7728
ISBN 0-394-48049-X

Manufactured in the United States of America

FIRST EDITION

To the best there is—
my husband Neil Schachter

Contents

Diagrams have been drawn specially for this book by Leslie Sherwin.

Author's Note
and Acknowledgments

Brand-name cosmetics are referred to in this book primarily to help the reader identify the kind of product which is being discussed. Although I have selected them on the basis of effectiveness, availability, and moderate price, there are many others that are equally as good.

I have personally tried all the cosmetics and toiletries mentioned and have not suffered any allergic response. However, individual reactions vary. You should patch-test any new preparation in the manner described on pages 229–30. Remember, too, that homemade preparations do not have preservatives in them and will not last as long as store-bought cosmetics; they should also be kept under refrigeration.

Many people gave generously of their time and knowledge to help make this book possible. I would especially like to thank Dr. Dicran Goulian, chief of plastic surgery at New York Hospital, Cornell Medical Center; Dr. Ivan Cohen, practicing dermatologist, New Haven; and Dr. Robert Sherwin, attending physician in endocrinology at Yale School of Medicine, New Haven. I am also deeply grateful to my mother, Martha Chase, whose care of my daughter, Karen, gave me the precious time to write; my father, Allan Chase, who took time off from his own book to work with me; Leslie Sherwin, whose exquisite illustrations complement and clarify the text; and my editor, Regina Ryan, who worked nights and weekends to shape a rough manuscript into a finished book. A special appreciation goes to my husband Neil—despite a heavy schedule as resident at Bellevue Hospital, New York, he did everything from reviewing the text for medical accuracy to shopping for dinner. Without his support the book would have remained a two-page outline.

Introduction

This book has been designed to give the average woman the hows and whys of beauty care that have long been known to physicians and cosmetic chemists.

Although this is not a book on science, it does offer, in everyday language, many of the factual, no-nonsense answers science has provided for some of the common beauty questions, such as:

> What causes dry skin?
>
> What causes hair to grow in gray?
>
> What is the difference between paste, cream, and liquid shampoos?
>
> How does a facial astringent work?
>
> Are there different kinds of acne? And, if so, how should each be treated?
>
> Do facial exercises help wrinkles?
>
> What does menopause do to a woman's skin and hair?
>
> Why does a conditioner make dull hair shiny?
>
> Can birth control pills help your skin?
>
> What is dandruff and what can be done about it?
>
> How does a face mask act on the skin?
>
> Which is the best night cream for lines?
>
> Do the words "hypo-allergenic" on the label of a beauty product mean anything? And, if so, what?

The people who are best trained to answer these and hundreds of other beauty questions that are dealt with in this book—the dermatologists, internists, endocrinologists, plastic surgeons, and cosmetic chemists—quite properly see themselves as physicians and scientists and not as cosmetologists. However, precisely because they are occupied with the responsibilities of helping seriously ill people or studying basic science, the field of beauty advice is frequently left to self-trained cosmeticians and sales people at retail counters and to the imaginative advertising copy writers who compose the print, radio, and television advertisements for cosmetics and other beauty products. Their answers to the spoken and unspoken beauty questions of upward of a hundred million American women are designed to sell specific products. This they do, even if the same products prove to be scientifically unsound, functionally worthless, and highly overpriced.

Today, women invest hundreds of dollars and thousands of hours annually in the relentless pursuit of beauty and good grooming. In 1970 alone, according to the U.S. Department of Commerce, American women spent a total of fourteen billion dollars on cosmetics and other beauty aids.

As various consumer-oriented books have shown in recent years, much of this money is spent on scandalously overpriced products and procedures whose claims are often spurious and which can sometimes be disfiguring. On the other hand, many commercial products and new grooming techniques can be of real value. This book sorts through much of the current beauty literature, separating fact from fantasy, to provide women with an accurate, easy-to-understand manual of total beauty care.

Essentially, this book is a manual of beauty care, based on the best and most advanced medical knowledge available today. It is not meant to be a challenge to the cosmetic or beauty care industries. Parts of this book, however, do run contrary to the established, popular, and often dated ideas of beauty care, some of which are widely promoted by the cosmetic, appliance, and beauty establishments.

The last fifty years have been a time of vast increases in new knowledge in biology and medicine. In fact, 90 percent of all modern scientific knowledge has been acquired since the end of World War I. But far too few of the revolutionary advances in the medical and other sciences are currently reflected in the day-to-day grooming ideas and practices of the average woman. The cosmetic industry has barely scratched the surface of the useful scientific knowledge available. For many reasons, chiefly economic, manufacturers are unwilling to invest the often enormous amounts of time and money in the basic research required to come up with a truly revolutionary face cream, soap, or hair conditioner. Since profit is the moving force behind the cosmetic industry, as in every other industry, success goes to those companies that sell the most goods, and to most manufacturers this means that success lies in turning out the most appealing, marketable products at the lowest possible production costs. By and large, while the packaging has grown fancier and the advertising costlier, the average line of beauty products on the market today derives from formulas and grooming techniques developed around the turn of this century—and earlier.

For example, the concept of facial massage flourished in the early 1900's. In its time, it was considered a revolutionary, scientific approach to skin care. That was also a time when there were no antibiotics; when tuberculosis was a major cause of death; diabetes and pneumonia were nearly always fatal diseases; and there were no polio, diphtheria, measles, whooping cough, and rubella vaccines. Today, in the era of organ transplants, open-heart surgery, and hormone therapy, we have new knowledge of skin and muscle biology that proves facial massage to cause far more harm than good; yet this out-of-date technique is still stubbornly held to be a valuable beauty aid.

Some cosmetic techniques used today are even older than facial massage. Various animal and vegetable oils were used to soften their skins by the women of Egypt over five thousand years ago. The formula for cold cream was invented in A.D. 200 by Galen, the Roman physician, and it is still the basis for many beauty creams used today.

The current fad for cosmetics compounded of herbs is based on the herbal knowledge of early sixteenth-century Europe—an era when the life span of the average human being was less than half as long as it is today in America and Europe.

With what has been learned about skin biology and chemistry in even the past twenty years, it seems shameful to continue to rely on old formulas and concepts that owe as much to witchcraft and superstition as they do to practical knowledge, let alone science.

Most of the research dollar of the cosmetic industry goes into the problems of manufacturing and packaging the same old products. Cosmetic executives are primarily concerned with the chemical problems of keeping emulsions stable, the engineering problems of preparing huge batches of soap, or the physical problems of preventing the discoloration of a beauty product as it sits on a store shelf.

Because they feel women are easily bored by last year's beauty preparation (possibly because the women are weary of it not working as promised), they are perpetually introducing new products. These new items will often be almost identical in formula to the older products they replace, differing only in their new "image"—a quality created solely by advertising writers, not by cosmetic chemists. They will, naturally, be marketed in entirely new containers, and launched with dazzingly new and novel advertising themes: The sun-dappled country girl in blue jeans; the "Cosmo" super swinger with a plunging neckline, or the elegantly groomed young matron.

When a formula works well in one form, cosmetic chemists are assigned to see if the same formula can be put up as a lotion, gel, ointment, cream, aerosol spray, soap, or milky cleanser. They thin it out; put it in a spray; add vitamins to one formula, sea salts to another. They take out the perfumes and call it hypo-allergenic. They put in extracts of cucumbers or strawberries and call it organic.

The number of creams, lotions, soaps, and masks becomes endless. One medium-sized manufacturer offers, for dry skin, in just one series of its multiple line of products, five cleansers, three astringents, thirteen creams and lotions, and two face masks.

Not all traditional cosmetics, of course, are out of date, and there have been some valuable advances in the qualities and the benefits of many commercial beauty products. One of the major aims of this book is to guide the woman through this labyrinth of beauty products and techniques to take sensible advantage of twentieth-century biology and medicine.

It will acquaint her with the ingredients of these cosmetics, and evaluate them in terms of her own individual beauty and grooming problems. A woman will be able, with the help of this book, to create her own programs of skin and hair care, and learn what practices and products to avoid.

Women today are better educated and better informed than ever before. They have the intelligence to understand the scientific and medical facts of beauty care and deserve better than the misconceptions and half truths that now pass for beauty knowledge. *The Medically Based No-nonsense Beauty Book* will give her just such information.

June 1974   D.C.

Part One / The Skin

1 / What the Skin Is Made of and How It Grows

Almost everyone is born with a beautiful complexion—velvety smooth, without visible pores or splotches, little red veins, lines, or wrinkles—radiant with good health. However, within fifteen years, all sorts of problems, such as oily skin, blackheads, pimples, and large pores, arise. Then just when these adolescent difficulties seem to be resolving, along come dry skin, wrinkles, baggy skin around the eyes, and brown spots.

Most women want to correct these and any other skin problems that may plague them. To be successful in the fight against the new insults the skin seems to dream up every day, a women has to understand her skin—what it is made of, how it gets its nourishment, what it needs to flourish and look wonderful. In short, a woman needs to understand the biology and chemistry of her skin.

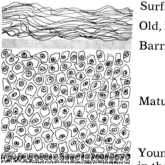

EPIDERMIS

Surface of the Skin

Old, Dead Cells

Barrier Level

Mature Cells

Young New Color
in the Base Layer

Diagram 1. A schematic view of the four major layers of the epidermis.

The skin is made up primarily of two layers, the *epidermis* and the *dermis* (see Diagram 1). The epidermis, the topmost layer, shows all the skin problems. This is the part that blisters, scales, discolors, gets splotches and pimples. The dermis lies below the epidermis, and in addition to supporting and nourishing the epidermis it contains such important structures as the oil and sweat glands, the hair follicles, and the blood vessels, all of which, in addition to being important in the skin's appearance, contain the reasons for many of the problems of the epidermis.

The Epidermis

The epidermis is built in layers and each layer has a different function.

The lowest layer, called the *basal layer*, is where the cells of the epidermis are born. These are plump healthy cells that reproduce rapidly, and gradually rise to the surface. These cells lie right next to the dermis, with its rich supply of blood vessels and glandular secretions. Their health and growth is dependent on the food and oxygen that the tiny capillaries (blood vessels) of the dermis carry. The same capillaries dispose of most of the cell's waste products, such as carbon dioxide.

If the circulation through these blood vessels is sluggish, less oxygen and nourishment are available to the basal layer, and more carbon dioxide and wastes remain in the cells. As a result, the cells of the basal layer do not grow and divide as rapidly as they normally do. Decreased circulation to all parts of the body occurs to some extent with aging, particularly after fifty, and this condi-

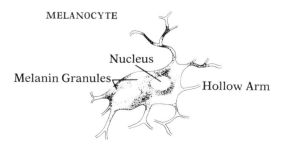

Diagram 2. *The melanocyte uses its hollow arms to "inject" melanin granules into the skin cells.*

tion is one of the factors in the decline of skin tone and appearance.

A few of the cells in the basal layer become *melanocytes*, the cells that give the brown color to skin by producing a chemical compound (or pigment) known as *melanin*. At first, these cells look just like any other cell, round and flat with a dark spot in the center called the nucleus, making it look rather like a fried egg. But the cells destined to become melanocytes begin to change. They develop long, hollow arms or extensions projecting out of their sides (see Diagram 2). These cells contain *enzymes* that under the proper conditions lead to the production of melanin. Then, using their hollow arms, the melanocytes take hold of a neighboring skin cell and inject the melanin into them.

Sunlight increases the production of melanin, giving light-skinned people the characteristic brown hue of a suntan. Bleaching creams, which lighten the skin, act by breaking down melanin.

As noted earlier, the cells of the basal layer are pushed up into the other layers. As they move upward they undergo many changes. One of the most important changes is the increase in the amount of *keratin*, a cell-produced protein substance, within the cells.

By the time the cells of the basal layer reach the top layer of the epidermis they are no longer alive, and they are entirely formed of keratin. This process of growth, maturation, and death is called *keratinization*. Problems in the speed and amount of keratin formation, as well as of its disposal, lead to many skin problems such as thickened, cracked, and even infected skin.

If the cells contain too little keratin, the appearance of the skin changes. It becomes cracked and flaky and cells slough off. This can leave the lower layers exposed to infection and irritation. Keratin needs water to keep it pliable and healthy. When the skin's water content decreases, the keratin crumbles, and the cells can't stay together. This is what is happening when the skin becomes dry.

The water level of the skin is dependent primarily on the third layer of the epidermis, called the *barrier level* (see Diagram 1). The cells in this layer are very thin, and they make up a membrane that controls the flow of water and oxygen into the skin and the evaporation and disposal of water and carbon dioxide out of the skin.

The barrier level is thought to contain a group of water-attracting compounds called Natural Moisturizing Factors, or

N.M.F.'s for short: Many doctors feel these compounds play a major role in maintaining a healthy water level in the skin.

As a man or woman grows older the amount of N.M.F. present in the skin decreases, which is one of the reasons that skin becomes dry with advancing age. Fortunately, N.M.F.'s have recently been synthesized (manufactured in laboratories) and are now commercially available in a few products.

The uppermost layer of the epidermis, layer 4 (see Diagram 1), is made up of old dried cells, which tend to be hard and brittle. These cells are primarily composed of keratin and do not reproduce. Their main function is to protect the layers lying directly beneath. Coating this layer are the waste products of the skin, in particular old sweat and stale oil, as well as the waste products of cellular metabolism. This could be considered the dumping ground of the skin.

The dead upper layer is meant to be removed; in fact, its removal actually stimulates cell growth in the lower layers. If it is not removed by proper washing the skin looks dull and muddy. The accumulated waste products plug up the pores and cause blackheads and pimples.

In normal skin, thorough cleansing will remove the right amount of the topmost layer. With oily skin, the oil tends to make the layer 4 cells more difficult to remove, because these cells stick together and special treatment is needed. On the other hand, dry skin makes the cells loose, and too many cells may be removed by normal washing.

The Acid Mantle

The acid mantle is a fluid that bathes the top layer of the skin. It is composed of fresh sebum (the secretion of the oil gland), sweat, and dissolved secretions from cells. It is believed that it acts as a natural defense barrier against skin infection. The fluid is acid; this means that it possesses certain chemical characteristics. Anything that radically changes the acidity of this fluid can result in beauty problems.

When skin is healthy, it will have a good acid mantle. Within one to three hours after the application of mildly alkaline substances, such as most face creams, the skin will return to its naturally acid state. With stronger alkalies, such as soap, it will take the skin longer to resume its normal acid balance.

The care of the acid mantle is most important for oily and acned skins. Without the acid mantle, these skins are more prone to bacterial infections, and it is particularly important that all products used for skin care be neutral or mildly acidic in nature. Both acned and oily skins require frequent washings, hence the proper *pH* (acid/alkaline balance) of the soap is all the more essential.

It is necessary to maintain the acid mantle while cleansing the skin thoroughly in order to keep the skin clear and smooth. Proper washing with a good soap will remove the dirt and grease without permanently interfering with the natural acid/alkaline balance of the skin.

The Dermis

While most of the skin's problems are seen on the epidermis, many of them are caused by troubles that originate below, in the dermis.

The dermis contains blood vessels, oil and sweat glands, and fat cells; it is held together by collagen. Problems with any of these parts can affect the skin's health and appearance.

Collagen

The dermis (see Diagram 3) is made up of collagen fibers (about 70 percent) that are arranged in regular patterns, like a

DERMIS

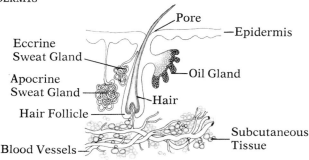

Diagram 3. The dermis lies below the epidermis, and many of the skin's problems begin here.

meshwork of nylon fibers, and that give the skin strength, form, and stability. These collagen fibers are produced by special cells found in the dermis.

Although many people think the general sagging of the skin in later years results from relaxation of facial muscles, and thus try to stimulate these muscles by exercise, electric shock, massage, or face masks, they could not be more wrong. It is the state of the skin's collagen, *not* that of the facial muscles, which determines how much the skin will wrinkle. When the collagen fibers lose their flexibility with age, the skin will wrinkle and sag because the underlying structure is gone.

Oil Glands

A second important component of the dermis is the oil gland. The oil glands are tiny coiled structures that lie next to the hair follicle (see Diagram 3). This gland has a little tube that connects with the hair follicle. As oil is produced by the cells of the gland, it travels down the tube into the follicle and is eventually pushed up and out of the pore onto the skin's surface. This oil spreads thinly and evenly over the skin, forming a protective coat.

The opening through which the oil flows onto the skin's surface is the tiny pore you see on the skin. The pore is of primary importance in many beauty problems. It can get clogged up with oil and acne eruptions will occur; the pore may become enlarged and obvious on the face; and, under certain conditions, it can produce dark coarse hairs.

The oil glands have probably more bearing on the appearance of the skin at any age than any other part of the skin. The main function of the oil is to supply a protective covering to insure that the skin retains the water it needs to be soft and smooth. The oil itself does not soften and smooth the skin, but acts as a shield against water evaporation. The oil covering simply guarantees that the water already present in the skin remains there.

Excess oil causes blackheads, pimples, and even cysts. Too little oil contributes to dry skin, and fine lines. The amount of oil produced depends on many factors—diet, medications, and heredity are only a few.

The oil glands are found primarily on the face, and to a lesser extent on the chest, back, and genital region. They are very sparse on the legs, arms, and stomach area. The skin on these parts of the body has to rely on the surface spreading of the oil from the oil-rich areas to the oil-poor ones. This transfer does not always function properly and one can frequently have oily skin on the face and dry skin on the legs and arms.

Sweat Glands

The sweat glands are also found in the dermis. There are two kinds of sweat glands, the *apocrine* and the *eccrine*. The apocrine glands are found under the arm, in the genital region, and in the nipples. They are tiny coiled structures connected to the hair follicles. They release their secretion through the same pores as the oil gland (see Diagram 3). Under emotional stress, such as fear, surprise, tension, or during intercourse, they secrete minute quantities of milky white fluid. When first released, this secretion is odorless. However, within a short period of time, the bacteria that are normally present on the skin's surface feed on the fats of this secretion, producing a pungent smell.

The eccrine sweat glands are far more numerous than the apocrine glands. They are found all over the body, and are especially prevalent on the forehead, the palms, and the soles of the feet. They are not connected to the hair follicle. They have their own duct and pores through which their secretions reach the skin's surface. When the body is subjected to a rise in temperature, such as on a hot day, or during physical exercise, the glands produce sweat. Unlike the sweat of apocrine glands, eccrine sweat does not become pungent. One frequently secretes from both the apocrine and eccrine glands at the same time.

This then is the skin—what it is made of and how it functions. All types of skin—dry, normal, oily, with special problems such as acne or excess hair—work the same way.

A few statements in this chapter contradict firmly held beauty beliefs, such as the relation of facial muscles to skin tone and wrinkles. These ideas, generally promoted and encouraged by cosmetic companies and beauticians, are frequently the result of ignorance, but more often than not they are generated to sell beauty products or treatments. This kind of misinformation makes it difficult to determine what kind of skin a woman really has, or how to treat it. For example, the beauty establishment works hard to convince women they have dry skin in order to sell them a huge array of creams, oils, and lotions. As a result, many women who have normal or even oily skin believe they have dry skin, and treat it with expensive creams and masks. This kind of treatment only makes their skin look much worse.

To correct this misinformation, the next chapter will explain the differences between the various soaps, creams, and astringents and indicate how to choose the best ones for your skin.

2 / The Basics
of Skin Care

Any skin, regardless of the problems it may have, requires three things: cleansing, oil-balance control, and toning.

Cleansing

Cleansing removes the outer layer of dead cells, stale oil, perspiration, and soot from the skin's surface. If this layer is not removed, the skin looks dull and flaky. The oil glands are blocked up and can start forming whiteheads and pimples, even in people with normally dry skin.

There is a huge array of products offered for cleansing— creams, lotions, and milky cleansers to name but a few. They all have different properties and should be used for different types of skin—some, in fact, should not be used at all.

Soap

Soap is the oldest and still the most common kind of cleanser. It was used as early as A.D. 200. By A.D. 700 soap makers' guilds had formed, and by 1700 the use of soap had spread to the remote corners of Europe.

The basic toilet soap consists of a mixture of fat, alkali salt, and water. Frequently coconut oil or palm kernel oil is added to give the soap better lathering properties. The basic formula of toilet soap has the ability to remove the dry dead cells that coat the skin's surface and the capacity to dissolve stale oil, sweat, and soot. Special ingredients are often added to give the soap unique properties.

KINDS OF SOAPS:

Superfatted soaps. They contain extra amounts of oils and fats. These are good for people with normal or slightly dry skin. The increased fat and oil content interferes with the soap's ability to remove oil efficiently. As a result, some oil remains on the face and the skin is less in danger of becoming dehydrated and dry.

Castile soap. It has olive oil as its main fat. It has no special properties. It is no less drying or richer than the basic toilet soap.

Transparent soap. It is made with the addition of glycerin and alcohol. It is widely promoted as a soap for dry skin. While it does leave a soft feeling on the skin after washing, it can be quite drying in the long run. Glycerin and alcohol both have the ability to draw water out of the skin, which, of course, dehydrates the skin, making it dry and flaky. In addition, transparent soap does not have enough degreasing strength for oily or acne-prone skins. People with normal skin, however, can use this kind of soap without any problem.

Deodorant soaps. They contain antibacterial chemicals. Hexachlorophene was the most common such chemical used before it was banned by the F.D.A. These chemicals kill the bacteria normally present on the skin's surface. Under normal circumstances these bacteria feed on the perspiration from the apocrine (sweat) glands, changing the sweat from an odorless liquid to its characteristic pungent state. Without the bacteria, the perspiration stays odorless. These soaps are good for the body, but have no special value when used on the face, where there are no apocrine glands.

French milled soaps. They have been specially processed to reduce their alkalinity. While a low alkalinity content makes the soap less drying to the skin, these soaps are much more expensive than other forms of low-alkaline soaps, such as Basis, Dove, Nivea, that are just as good or even better for dry skin.

Floating soaps. They contain extra water and have air trapped in them. The fact that the soap floats does not give it any special properties for the skin.

Detergent soaps. These are synthetic soaps. While detergents conjure up an image of harsh chemicals and simple soaps seem so much gentler and better for the skin, just the reverse is often true. It is easier for the cosmetic chemist to adjust the properties of a detergent to make it better for the skin. It can be made less alkaline, less dehydrating, better lathering, and less irritating than plain soap. Detergent soaps are often called "soapless soaps."

Soaps with fruit, vegetable, and/or herb extracts. These are very popular today. Without exception, these additives do not give unique properties to a soap. The value of these soaps depends on the other basic ingredients that make up the body of the soap.

The concept of having fresh fruit, vegetables, or herbs in a cosmetic is very appealing to the senses. These ingredients conjure up an image of natural health, freshness, and purity. However, any value these ingredients may possess in the way of vitamins or enzymes is completely destroyed in the manufacturing process. For example, take cucumber soap. The basic ingredients of this soap are no different than those of any other: fat, salts, and water. Cucumbers are living plants. If you take a fresh cucumber, even one grown without pesticides, and throw it into a vat of soap, it will quickly decompose and rot. Living plants have to be treated before they can be added to any cosmetic. The juice must be squeezed out, sterilized, and condensed. Alcohol and preservatives are then added to make the juices stable. Cucumber perfume is added to make the soap smell like the real thing, and green dye is put into the mixture to reinforce the idea of a fresh cucumber.

There is simply no good reason to buy a soap on the basis of the fruits, vegetables, or herbs it may contain.

Cocoa-butter soap. Cocoa butter is used to provide the basic fat ingredient in the soap. This fat does not give any unique property to the soap. In addition, cocoa oil has been associated with many skin allergies.

WASHING WITH SOAP: Whatever type of soap you choose, it should be worked up in a lather in your hands and spread on your already moistened face. It should be rubbed thoroughly all over your face and then rinsed off just as thoroughly. The rubbing motion on the face helps the soap loosen the dead cells and dissolve the grease.

Although people with normal or oily skin can use a washcloth to aid in the removal of oil and dead cells, a washcloth is too rough for dry skin. When washing the body, a natural sponge or bath brush will aid in the removal of dead skin cells.

Creams and Other Cleansers

COLD CREAMS: These are the simplest and most commonly used cleansing creams. They are made up of mineral oil, wax, and borax. When rubbed on the skin they dissolve the oils on the surface and loosen the superficial dead cells. When the cold cream is tissued off, the oil and cells are removed. However, cold cream leaves behind an oil film that contains some of the dirt that would have been removed by washing with soap. The skin does not get as clean as it would with soap.

CLEANSING CREAMS: These are made of wax, mineral oil, alcohol, water, and some kind of soap or detergent. These products are rubbed all over the face and the excess cream is tissued off. After such a treatment the skin often feels sticky and unclean and there is a good reason for this: the skin is not clean. The thick creams cannot create enough friction when rubbed on the skin to remove the dead cells. It makes them clump together and they remain on the skin's surface. In addition, the soap in these cleansing creams also remains in the film coating the skin. The soap damages the keratin and dries out the skin.

Because the skin feels so sticky after a cleansing cream, women often use a skin freshener with alcohol or another harsh solvent to remove this layer of grease. Not only do these products remove the remains of the cream but they also strip off all the existing natural skin oils. This type of cleanser does not do a satisfactory job of cleansing normal or oily skin. The remains of its soap film or the added insult of removal by a solvent may lead to devastating results for dry skin. This is one of the most heavily promoted types of cleansers, and one of the worst. It is not good for any type of skin.

CLEANSING LOTIONS: These are made of the same ingredients as cleansing creams, but contain more water. They have the same drawbacks as do the solid cleansing creams.

. . .

LIQUEFYING CLEANSING CREAMS: These have the same ingredients as the regular cleansing creams, but they are designed to melt at body temperature. This does not give the product any better cleansing properties, and again all the disadvantages of cleansing creams are present.

WASHABLE CREAMS: These are compounded of similar ingredients as those described above, but they have been formulated to make them water soluble. This means that after they are rubbed on the face, and have dissolved the stale oils and loosened dead cells, the cream may be washed off with water. The rinsing off of the cream removes any trace of soap along with the dirt. Washable creams do a thorough but gentle job of cleansing and are good for normal and dry skins, but they do not have enough degreasing power for oily skin.

MILKY CLEANSERS: These are a combination of soap, water, alcohol, and mineral oil. They contain more soap and less oil than do washable creams. They are really primarily soaps and are thereby good cleansers for normal and slightly oily skin. They are too harsh for dry skin.

SCRUBBING CLEANSERS: These are soaps containing tiny grains that act as an abrasive on the skin. These cleansers rub off the surface of the skin. A scrubbing cleanser should be used once weekly for normal skin and at least once daily on oily skin. It is an additional soap in the skin care program. It is not to be used every day as a regular cleanser unless oiliness is pronounced.

Oil-balance Control

Every type of skin, with the exception of oily and acned skin, needs some lubrication. The application of any oil or cream is used to create a better shield against water evaporation; it in effect supplements the skin's own natural shield. There are many products available for this purpose and they are intended for both day and night use.

. . .

Day Creams
and Daytime Lotions

Day creams are all designed to be worn under makeup. As such they must be nongreasy in order not to discolor the makeup. They supposedly prepare the skin to better accept a foundation. When applied, many seem to disappear into the skin. For this reason they are often called "vanishing creams." Actually these products do not penetrate deeply into the skin; rather they stay on the surface, spreading out in an imperceptible film on the very top layer. In fact, very few things go through the skin's layers. No cream or lotion can ever sink deeply into the skin, and certainly none of these products can "go deep into the skin to nourish and revitalize it" as so many creams and lotions claim.

Thick day creams are made basically of wax, water, oil, and a lot of soap. That's right, soap. The soap is necessary to make the cream thick and less greasy so that it does not dissolve makeup. These thick soapy creams are very bad for all types of skin, and should not be used.

Creamy daytime *lotions*, on the other hand, have the same ingredients as thick creams but contain more water and *much less* soap. These lotions frequently contain additional ingredients such as estrogen or synthesized Natural Moisturizing Factors (N.M.F.'s), which may help the skin maintain a better water balance. Because of the presence of these added chemicals, such products are frequently called *moisturizers*. They are excellent products for dry skin, but are unnecessary for normal or oily skin.

The general, all-purpose hand, body, and face lotion is made with four basic ingredients—water, wax, lanolin, and glycerin. It is frequently somewhat oilier than the undermakeup moisturizer, but it will not discolor makeup. It usually does not contain N.M.F.'s or other water-hungry chemicals. This lotion is inexpensive and it has many uses in beauty care routines.

The promotion of many creams relies heavily on the supposed value of the oils they contain. Peach kernel oil, mineral oil, lanolin, wheat-germ oil—which is best? This is a very important question to ask yourself when buying such a cosmetic. Many products command much higher prices because they contain such specific oils as turtle oil or apricot oil, which are supposed to leave your skin softer. Are these prices justified?

Oils may be divided into three categories:

1. Vegetable oils, such as corn, safflower, olive, wheat-germ, and all the nut oils.

2. Mineral oils, such as regular mineral oil or petroleum derivatives.

3. Animal fats, like codfish oil, lanolin (derived from sheep), mink oil, and turtle oil.

All these oils are meant to coat the skin and delay the evaporation of water. None has any special power to delay aging or prevent the formation of lines and wrinkles.

Of all the oils, animal fats, particularly *lanolin*, seem to do the best job. Lanolin and other animal fats most closely resemble the natural human sebum (oil). Not only do animal fats maintain the skin's water level but they also do not interfere with the skin's normal activities, such as sweating, breathing, and eliminating the natural waste products of the skin's rapidly growing cells. The most expensive animal fats—mink and turtle oil—are no better than lanolin, and their high prices are in no way justified. Mink oil is extracted from the scraps of minks discarded by furriers. Turtle oil has no special vitamins or anti-aging properties (turtles may live a long time, but it is not because of their oil). In its raw natural state turtle oil is foul-smelling and must be heavily processed before it can be used commercially.

Vegetable oils provide good coverage for the skin, but not quite as good as lanolin. Polyunsaturated oils (vegetable oils) are probably good in your diet, but on your skin they have no unique or magic powers. There is little difference in moisturizing ability among the various vegetable oils—simply because one oil is harder to extract or available in smaller quantities (e.g., apricot kernel) does not mean that it is any better than a more readily available oil (e.g., corn oil) when used on the skin.

Mineral oils are not as good as animal or vegetable oils, particularly for very dry skin. They have a tendency to dissolve the skin's own natural oil, and can thereby increase dehydration. Nevertheless, they are very bland and safe and are used as a base for many cosmetics.

. . .

Night Creams

More nonsense has been attached to *night creams* than to any other beauty product. They command truly incredible prices, with many of them reaching thirty dollars an ounce, or five times the cost of pure silver. There is absolutely nothing in these creams that can justify such prices. Although for items like art or real estate it is not unreasonable to expect more when you pay more, a higher price on a night cream (and most other cosmetics, for that matter) rarely guarantees a better product.

All night creams are meant to do one thing—to help the skin retain a better supply of water. They cannot rejuvenate the skin, prevent lines or wrinkles, reach deep down into the pores, or wake up sleepy complexions, as is so often promised by cosmetic advertisements. All night creams provide a shield against water evaporation, allowing the skin to build up a supply of water that makes the skin feel soft and smooth. Some night creams that contain estrogens or other water-hungry substances are thought to do a better job of holding water in the skin. However, these are frequently priced the same as those night creams not containing them. How estrogen creams and estrogen-like creams work and how to buy them are discussed in Chapter 3 in the section on dry skin.

Night creams are made up of wax, oils, water, and emulsifiers like soap or borax. They are usually much thicker and oilier than day creams since they are not worn under makeup. Many useless additives are often put into night creams, which are then promoted as having special beautifying properties. Among the more common ones are:

AMINO ACIDS: These are the building blocks of proteins and are a basic ingredient in virtually every part of the body. However, even though the skin is constantly in need of protein to regenerate itself, it can never absorb or utilize the foreign proteins or amino acids spread on its surface. The idea that they can help build more skin is something out of science fiction.

COLLAGEN: This is the structure in the dermis giving the skin its strength and flexibility. However, the chopped-up extract that is now incorporated into creams is cosmetically worthless. The strength of the collagen fiber lies in its ordered structure. These fibers are linked together in such a way that the skin can easily move and shift its contours. To think that ground-up, processed collagen can help skin tone is like trying to restore an amputated limb by spreading a cream that contains ground-up arms and legs on the stump.

EGGS: The lecithin (a fat compound) that occurs naturally in eggs is used as an emulsifier—that is to say, it keeps the cosmetic in cream form and does not let the water separate from the solid components of the cream. Other than this stabilizing property eggs, or, more precisely, lecithin, cannot work any miracles on the surface of the skin. The skin cannot absorb the protein, minerals, or vitamins found in eggs.

HONEY: Many mystical properties have been attached to honey, none of which has been proven to be justified. In fact, the presence of honey in a cream increases the chance that the cream will cause allergic reactions. The pollen present in the honey can cause nasal congestion and skin rashes in those people who are allergic to flowers, grasses, and other natural allergenic materials.

VITAMINS: Only vitamins A and D can be absorbed by the skin and thereby have an effect on the health of the skin. All other vitamins, including the much-heralded vitamin E, cannot pass through the very topmost layer of the skin's protective coat and therefore cannot in any way influence the skin's condition when applied to its surface.

Toning

All types of skin require toning. Toning makes the skin look firm, lively, poreless, and smooth. There are three basic cosmetic tools that permit this effect: toning lotions, masks, and saunas.

Toning Lotions

Toning lotions are applied after the skin is washed and dried, but before moisturizers and makeup are put on. Toning lotions can make the skin look firmer, reinforce a healthy coloring, and can temporarily appear to shrink pores.

Toning lotions come under many different names. Sometimes the products have different properties and in other cases the different names are applied to the same kind of substance. There are three basic types of toning lotions: skin fresheners, astringents, and clarifying lotions.

SKIN FRESHENERS: These are basically alcohol with various additives, such as herb extracts to give them "character" and camphor or menthol to give them "zing" (the tingling sensation that occurs after application). They make the skin feel cool and refreshed but can be irritating to all but the oiliest skins. They are used primarily as grease removers for oily skin problems and in removing the sticky residue of nonwashable cleansing creams. They may also be called freshening lotions or skin tonics.

ASTRINGENTS: These contain water and small amounts of alcohol, and aluminum salts. They have the special ability to make pores *seem* smaller. Once a pore is stretched it can never really be closed, even temporarily. The aluminum salts in astringents cause a slight puffiness or swelling of the skin around the pore, cutting it off from view.

Because of the vast array of fanciful names given to astringents and fresheners, it is often difficult to figure out which is which, and it is very important to choose the right one. Astringents are a much more effective pore closer than are skin fresheners, and are in general much healthier for all types of skin.

Confusion persists because most cosmetic companies do not list the ingredients on their labels, but this situation is rapidly changing. The F.D.A. has recently announced that by March 1975 all cosmetics must have their ingredients printed on the label. Some companies, including Almay and Revlon, are already labeling some of their products. Avon will frequently provide the list of ingredients for a cosmetic upon the request of a consumer. In the course of this book, the different ingredients to look for when you are buying a cosmetic are described. Then, if you wish, before you buy a new astringent, or any other beauty product you are interested in, you can write to the manufacturer for a list of ingredients. In the case of an astringent, if it contains an aluminum or zinc salt and fits the requirements listed below it will probably be a good astringent. If it does not, write to other manufacturers for the same type of product.

CLUES TO SELECTING THE MOST EFFECTIVE ASTRINGENT

1. Concentrate on products with "astringent" in the name. By definition, they are supposed to contain astringent substances—but beware, there is no *legal* definition of astringent so that there is no guarantee that you are really getting an astringent. Astringents are also called pore lotions.

2. Beware of really sharp stinging sensations. These prodducts probably contain only camphor or menthol (without any aluminum salts or alcohol); they often have a smell of peppermint. In their place they are good cosmetic aids—they jolt the circulation in the skin and give the skin a nice rosy glow. They are called *rubefactants* (*rube* meaning "red" and *factant* meaning "to cause"). But to hide the pores you want an astringent, not a rubefactant, which will not do as good a job.

3. Beware of products that are advertised to remove makeup. They have to contain chemicals that dissolve grease and makeup and cannot concentrate on pore-shrinking properties.

If you are still unsure about getting the most effective astringent, you can add alum (a type of aluminum salt) to a skin freshener or toner best for your type of skin (see Chapter 3, sections on normal, dry, or oily skin). Alum is used in the canning of fruits and vegetables and is available on the spice rack in the supermarket at about fifteen cents an ounce. One half a teaspoon of alum added to eight ounces of freshener will make an excellent astringent. If your freshener is really an astringent, the extra alum will not make it too strong.

CLARIFYING LOTIONS: These are the third and last type of toning lotion, and are meant to make the skin look brighter and clearer by taking off the top layer of dry dead cells. They contain water, alcohol, glycerin, and a chemical that can dissolve keratin, which makes up most of the skin's top layer. These substances are called *keratolytic agents*, meaning simply that they break down keratin. Chemicals that are keratolytic include salicylic acid, resorcinol, and benzyl peroxide. If present in a cosmetic these three substances must by law be listed on the container's label. Papain, an enzyme extracted from papayas, and bromelin, an enzyme extracted from pineapples, can also dissolve keratin. These two substances do not have to be listed on the label of the product in which they appear, although they are very powerful keratolytic agents and have been associated with allergies and chemical burns.

Clarifying lotions may also be formulated to be extremely alkaline or may have a high alcohol content. Both alkaline substances or alcohol can remove the topmost keratin layer, but these will more often than not damage healthy skin in addition to removing the dry dead skin cells. In some instances a clarifying lotion may simply contain a standard astringent, with no special keratolytic agent. If so, it is not truly a clarifying lotion. Unfortunately, there is no law that says that a cosmetic has to live up to its promises.

Many clarifying lotions do not have any ingredients on the label. These may well contain papain or bromelin or even some other unregulated keratolytic chemicals, so it is safer to buy one that has the keratolytic agents listed.

If there are no ingredients listed, write the manufacturer, asking what chemical or types of chemicals form the active keratolytic agent of the product.

Clarifying lotions are also known as *exfoliating lotions*.

Masks

Masks come in two basic forms—*clay* and *gel*. Clay masks asbsorb excess oil and dirt from the skin. They pick up the cellular debris and give the skin a smooth, even texture. As the mask dries, the tightening action stimulates circulation, and makes the skin glow. The clay itself contains mild bleaching agents that cause a gentle lightening of the skin. The clay also smooths the skin, reducing the inflammation and soreness. Finally, a clay mask acts as a complete barrier against evaporation, allowing the skin to store up a large supply of water for as long as it remains on the skin.

Gel masks are made of a clear gel that is usually supplied in a tube. It is spread on the face and allowed to dry. After drying, it is pulled off in one piece. This type of mask is especially good for restoring water or rehydrating normal, normal/dry, and dry skin. It does not soak up oil, but its solid, stretched film encourages the skin to store up water. At the same time it gives a gentle boost to the circulation while it dries and hardens. When the mask is pulled off the face it takes with it the loose flaky skin on the surface.

Most of a mask's value lies in the clay or gel base that forms the mask itself, although you can get special effects by adding certain ingredients. Many commercial masks have strange and exotic ingredients that don't do a thing—such as strawberries, sea salts, herbs, and honey. Some additives, however, increase the beauty value of a mask and it is important to find out which ones they are. For example, estrogens, N.M.F.'s, and silicones increase the water retention of the skin. Masks are often very expensive and you do not want to pay for useless ingredients. Check the glossary for the potential value of other additives that may be present.

Saunas

Saunas are marvelous for every type of skin. The warm, moist heat loosens the skin's top dried layer so that it can be removed, melts clogged-up oil in the pores, stimulates circulation, and provides a lot of water for the skin.

The electric facial sauna comes in a wide price range, from a low of eight dollars to a high of three hundred dollars. Most of them do very much the same thing; they bathe the face in gentle steam. Some are "designed" to be used with herbs or other additives to the water. This does *not* improve their value.

Just as efficient is the sauna that can be made at home with a pot of hot water and a towel.

Fill a large pot with water and bring to a boil. Carry the pot to a steady table. Sit down in front of the steaming pot and drape a towel over your head and shoulders to envelop you and the pot in a towel tent. This is a very hot sauna, much hotter than a commercial sauna, and you might find you have to lift the towel and get a couple of gulps of fresh, cool air during the sauna period. *Be sure to keep your face at least a foot away from the steaming pot* (and keep the children out of the room).

Examine your skin after five to ten minutes under the facial sauna. See how plump and smooth the skin is—lines seem to disappear and the skin feels very soft. This demonstrates vividly the effect simple water has on the beauty of the skin.

The Care of Body Skin

Cleansing, oil-balance control, and toning are the basics of facial skin care. Body skin, while very much like facial skin, has some differences and requires a few additional products. Primarily, these are substances added to your bath (there are three kinds of bath additives: bath salts, bath oils, and bubble baths); body powders and lotions; as well as anti-perspirants and deodorants.

BATH SALTS: These are designed primarily to soften hard water—water that contains large quantities of minerals. Soap does not clean well in hard water; it refuses to lather and remains on the body and hair as a dry sticky film. Bath salts remove the excess minerals present in hard water and thereby make this water more suitable for bathing. Bath salts consist of a salt, like sodium carbonate, mixed with perfume and a dye. These products are frequently alkaline and can be drying to the skin.

There is a kind of bath salt that is supposed to be an aid in reducing fat. This "special" formula contains very large quantities of salts that, in a warm bath, can cause a temporary weight loss by encouraging the skin to give up water. One or two hours after such a bath, the body restabilizes its water level and the weight, alas, returns.

BATH OILS: These contain water, a soap (or detergent), a perfumed oil, and frequently a small amount of alcohol. They leave an oil film on the body that softens the skin and cuts down on the evaporation of water. Bath oils are often used by dermatologists for the care of a wide variety of itchy dry-skin problems.

BUBBLE BATHS: These are made with a sulfur-derivative detergent, water, perfume, and artificial coloring. Some long-lasting bubble baths contain substances that stabilize the bubbles and make them stronger. Bubble baths have a pleasant, calming psychological effect. They do not, in general, soften either your bath water or your skin. The sulfur-based detergents can irritate the delicate tissues of the vagina.

BATH POWDERS: These are patted on the body after a bath and serve to absorb excess moisture. They prevent chafing in the body creases, especially during hot weather. They are composed of talc, chalk, perfume, and coloring.

BODY LOTIONS: These are the all-purpose lotions described earlier, on page 16, and are used on the face and body, day or night, to lubricate normal and slightly dry skin.

ANTI-PERSPIRANTS AND DEODORANTS: These are the most commonly used toiletries today. Anti-perspirants are made of water and aluminum salts; they are very similar in composition to facial astringents, and act on the same principles. Aluminum salts in these products cause the skin surrounding the sweat glands to puff up around the pore opening. This stops the flow of perspiration out of the sweat ducts. Aluminum salts are considered active ingredients by the F.D.A. and must therefore be listed on the label.

Deodorants do not stop the sweat glands from perspiring, but act by interfering in some way with the growth of bacteria on the skin. Some contain substances that kill the bacteria; others, in addition to killing the bacteria, contain chemicals that make the skin inhospitable to further bacterial growth. A third kind of deodorant does not destroy bacteria, but simply prevents them from acting on the perspiration to cause odor.

This chapter has explained the basics of cosmetics. The next section will go into more detail about determining what kind of skin you have, choosing the products for your skin's needs, and setting up a successful beauty care program.

3 / Typing and the Care of Your Skin

One of the keys to caring successfully for skin is correctly naming the type of skin you have.

The face you see in the mirror at this moment does not necessarily tell the whole story. It has been subjected to many creams, lotions, mud packs, and soaps. Its true condition may have been disguised for such a long time that you may not know what kind of skin you really have. For example, a skin that looks very dry could really be normal skin that has been dried out too much by soaps and harsh treatments.

To discover what skin type you really have, think back on the history of your skin. What kind of skin did your parents have? What color is your hair? Are you fair- or olive-complexioned? All of these factors are important to the present and future state of your skin.

Here are a series of profiles to determine if you have normal, dry, or oily skin. The profile that most accurately describes your skin gives a good clue to the best program of treatment for you. For the discussion of normal skin, see pages 28–34; for dry skin, pages 35–44; for oily skin, pages 44–50.

A PROFILE OF NORMAL SKIN

1. Did you have mild acne as a teenager? Did it respond to a soap, drying lotion, and diet program of care? Did it begin when you were about fifteen and pretty much disappear by the time you were eighteen or nineteen?

2. Do your parents both have good skin?—that is, they don't have problems with acne, nor do they have deep acne scars.

3. Do you wash your hair about twice a week? After three or four days does it get a bit oily? Not greasy, just dull and flat?

4. Are you free of obvious facial hair above your mouth or on your cheeks?

5. For four days, stop using all your regular cosmetics. Wash twice daily with a mild neutral soap like Dove (Lever Brothers) or Basis (Duke). Use no creams, masks, or powders. (You can use eye makeup.) Now look at your skin critically. Does it feel smooth? Does it remain fairly clean during the day? Is there a nice translucent glow rather than an oily sheen?

6. Do you have few or no enlarged pores?

7. Is the color even? (There should be no reddish patches, which give the skin a splotchy, irritated look.)

8. If you are between twenty to thirty-five years old, are there any signs of real dryness—that is, flaky skin on the cheeks or nose? (Flaky skin on the forehead and chin generally is a sign of too harsh a cleansing.)

9. If very cold or dry weather dehydrates the skin, making it chapped, can mild creams and lotions quickly restore your skin to its original fresh appearance?

10. Do you tan easily?

11. Does your makeup foundation remain in fairly good shape for a whole day without caking or with no oily shine breaking through?

A PROFILE OF DRY SKIN UNDER 30

1. Did you have an almost totally acne-free adolescence?

2. Do you have dry hair?

3. Is your skin smooth, unlined, yet "tight" even several hours after washing?

To qualify for youthful dry skin you should really answer yes to all three questions. If there is some doubt that these signs properly describe your skin, then it is very possible that you do not have true youthful dry skin, and to treat it as such will not achieve the best results.

A PROFILE OF DRY SKIN OVER 30

1. Does the surface of the skin feel dry and chapped?

2. Does your skin look raw and reddened?

3. Are there lines along your mouth, on your forehead, and around your eyes?

4. Does your skin look dull, thick, or coarse?

5. Does your skin ever get so chapped and dry that cracks appear on the surface?

A PROFILE OF OILY SKIN

1. Was your adolescent acne moderate to severe but did it respond fairly well to the conventional treatment?

2. After nineteen or twenty, was the acne limited to a few bumps each month? Did patches of small reddish spots sometimes appear along the jaw, which looked more like a rash than pimples, but were pimples?

3. Is your hair oily? Must it be washed frequently (three to four times per week) in order to look attractive?

4. Several hours after putting on makeup, does the face seem shiny?

5. Is there an oily film on the face in the morning, especially on the forehead, nose, and chin?

Normal Skin

Many people have normal skin but refuse to believe it. They are more or less dermal hypochondriacs. To such people, a slight tightness after washing means "dry skin!" and they slather their faces with oils and creams. To others, one pimple a month equals "terminal acne!" so they dry their faces with lotions and soaps to the consistency of old leather.

Many skin problems are due to mistakes in diagnosing the kind of skin a person has and then treating the skin for the wrong problems. For example, many young women between the ages of twenty and thirty feel they have a very difficult type of skin problem, described in cosmetic ads as "combination skin." They think they have dry skin, and yet are subject to pimples especially around the mouth and chin. Actually "combination skin" is frequently the result of using too many greasy creams and moisture lotions. Looking in the mirror, these women see flaky skin that looks dull and coarse. They think it is dry and rough, but they are wrong.

These women have normal or even oily skin, but have abused their skins unwittingly, by not removing the topmost layer of epidermis correctly. What they see is *caking*, not flaking, of the skin. Soap and water would take off this congealed skin, but the treatment usually recommended is moisture creams to smooth away the "dry skin." The pores, already struggling under a load of dead cells, cannot manage this oily onslaught and rebel with a blossoming of pimples.

This kind of mistreatment is not rare. In fact, about half of all acne found in this age group is caused by this common misconception. A few weeks of cleansing with a mild, neutral soap will go a long way toward clearing up this skin problem.

The point is that looking in the mirror, this girl would never believe she has normal skin. But she does, and the profile would have proved it. So if you have qualified for normal skin, read on and find out why your skin is healthy and how to keep it that way.

What Normal Skin Looks Like

Normal skin is very healthy skin. The oil glands secrete enough oil to prevent water evaporation from the skin, but not enough to plug up its pores and thereby cause acne and dilated or enlarged pores. The proper amount of oil gives the skin its attractive smooth sheen.

The attractive rosy color of normal skin indicates that the blood circulation through the dermis is good, and that the blood contains plenty of iron-rich hemoglobin. Good color also indicates that the top layer is thin and smooth enough to let the rosy color of the blood shine through, but not so thin that it appears rough, sore, and flaky.

With normal skin there will be no obvious dark facial hair, nor will there be splotches of red indicating easily irritated or sensitive skin.

In short, normal skin is balanced skin. All the biological processes are in perfect equilibrium with one another; the growth and death of cells are properly balanced. The right number of top cells (the upper layer of the epidermis) are flaking off to help keep the skin soft and fresh, and the right amount of new cells are born in the bottom (basal) layer. These new cells are healthy and vigorous and grow at a good, even rate.

The chemistry of normal skin is also balanced. It has enough N.M.F.'s to attract and keep water in the tissues; on its surface, the acid mantle is busily fighting off infection, and, in the dermis, the collagen is flexible and strong.

All normal skins, however, are not alike. There is no absolute amount of oil that should be produced, and no exact quota of cells that must fall off each hour. Rather, there is a range of normal activities in the skin.

Some normal skins might be a little dry, others a bit oily. However, when viewed as a whole, these skins are well balanced and healthy, and the key to keeping and perfecting normal skin lies in maintaining this balance.

The Care of Normal Skin

As you will recall from Chapter 2, on the basics of skin care, there are three basic steps to the care of any skin: cleansing, oil-balance control, and toning.

CLEANSING: Proper cleansing is the mainstay of normal skin. The right kind of cleansing will remove the stale oil, dirt, and dry dead cells to make the complexion look bright and clear, but will not remove too much water, which would cause the skin to look dry and flaky. There are three programs of cleansing that are good for normal skin: soap alone, plain cream followed by soap, and washable cleansing creams or lotions.

Soap. A well-compounded plain soap will do an excellent

job on normal skin, especially if little or no makeup is worn over it. The soap should be unscented, undyed (no color additives), super-fatted, and neutral in pH. Products that fit these qualifications are BASIS, NIVEA, and DOVE.

If you use a lot of eye makeup, but little or no makeup elsewhere on the face, remove the eye makeup with a cold cream and clean the rest of the face with soap and water. If you wear a good bit of makeup and your skin is never oily, then you might want to try the next cleansing method.

Cream and soap. This method involves cleansing the face first with a plain cold cream or solidified mineral oil such as ALBOLENE CREAM. After removing most of the cream with a tissue, the face is then washed with a mild neutral soap as before. Soap alone cannot dissolve heavy makeup, and cream alone cannot properly remove the top layer of skin, but a combination of the two is excellent for normal skin. It is totally unnecessary to get a cream with special ingredients like herbs or vitamins. It is on the face for too short a period of time for any of the additives to act.

Washable cleansing creams or lotions. An equally good and somewhat quicker method for removing makeup entails the use of washable creams or lotions. These products, which you rub around the face, then rinse off with water, are really a mixture of soap and cream. They have much less oil than regular cleansers, yet retain the same ability to dissolve makeup and oil. They also pick up the top layer of dead cells much more efficiently than standard creams. The rinsing used to remove them carries away the dissolved oil, the dead cells, and the residue of cleanser, leaving the skin clean, smooth, and soft. An example of this type of product is HAPPY FACE by Tussy.

Washable lotions, usually called beauty milks or milky cleansers, are made of the same ingredients as washable creams; however, they contain a good deal more water. Two examples of this product type are MILKY CLEANSER by Elizabeth Arden and ULTIMA II MILK BATH by Revlon.

SPECIAL CLEANSING: People with normal skin should use scrubbing soaps once weekly, preferably during the facial described at the end of this chapter. These soaps contain abrasive grains that remove the top layer of dead cells and the skin's grease very efficiently. Two products of this type are PERNOX and BRASIVOL.

OIL-BALANCE CONTROL: Normal skin needs very little help in the way of oil-balance control. The fact that it is normal means that the oil glands are producing sufficient oil to maintain the skin's water balance. However, indoor heating, air-conditioning, pollution, and cold windy weather can dehydrate even normal skin.

The best products to use at these times are light, plain, all-purpose lotions. These should contain considerable water, some oil, preferably lanolin or another animal oil, and should not contain perfume or dyes. Two products of this type are LUBRIDERM and NIVEA.

TONING: After the face is clean, the next step is to make the skin look firm, poreless, and smooth. To this end there are three types of products: astringents, masks, and saunas.

Astringents. This beauty aid, as described in the basic chapter on skin care, makes a pore seem smaller by puffing up the skin around it, cutting the pore off from view. Astringents get their special punch from aluminum salts (such as alum). As mentioned earlier, it is very difficult simply by reading the name of a product to differentiate which ones are truly astringents, and therefore contain such salts, and which are simply solutions of water, alcohol, and/or glycerin, with perfumed scent and a dye. These latter products are variously called pore lotions, skin fresheners, skin tonics, or even astringents.

To get around this dilemma, people with normal skin should buy any such named product, preferably one that is on sale, and add your own alum. As mentioned earlier, even if the product has alum in it, a little more won't hurt you. Alum is available on the spice rack in the supermarket. For a good, effective astringent, add one half a teaspoonful of alum to eight ounces of fluid. The astringent should be poured on a fresh cotton ball and rubbed lightly on the face, taking care not to rub it in the eyes. It should be allowed to dry on the skin before anything else is applied. Two products for normal skin to which alum can be added to make a good astringent are VELVA SMOOTH LOTION by Arden and DEEP MIST TONING AND REFINING LOTION by Almay.

Masks. Both clay and gel masks have their place in the care of normal skin.

Clay masks are useful for deep-cleansing and to remove oil and dirt.

Gel masks are excellent when cold winds, overheated rooms, or too much sun have dried out your usually normal skin.

A clay-based mask for normal skin is VELVA CREAM by Elizabeth Arden. Two gel masks for normal skin are Shiseido's FACIAL PACK and DEEP MIST GENTLE GEL MASK by Almay.

Saunas. The moist heat of the sauna dissolves stale oil, loosens the upper layer of dead cells, and feeds a nice supply of water to the skin, keeping it soft and smooth. People with normal skin should use a sauna once a week, preferably as part of a weekly facial.

Makeup and Normal Skin

People with normal skin can wear any kind of makeup. This type of skin has enough natural health to resist the effects of too oily or too drying cosmetics. Properly taken care of, normal skin will always look well.

A PROGRAM OF CARE FOR NORMAL SKIN

NIGHT

1. Cleanse according to preference. Be sure to wash with hot water.

2. Do not use an astringent at night.

3. Apply a small amount of the all-purpose lotion on your cheeks and forehead. Avoid the nose and chin, where the many oil glands supply enough oil to keep the skin smooth.

DAY

1. Cleanse as you did in the evening.

2. Apply an astringent with a small cotton ball. Use a fresh one each day—let your face dry.

3. Apply your makeup. Do *not* use an undermakeup moisturizer. Normal skin does not need a layer of cream under makeup. It will only clog up its pores and make the skin dull from congealed oil and dead cells. The oil present in most foundations gives normal skin more than enough lubrication. A foundation will remain fresher and cleaner on

normal skin without an underlying cream. If you are not going to wear any makeup, you can put on a small amount of all-purpose lotion if your skin seems a bit dry and/or if it's cold and windy weather.

WEEKLY DEEP-CLEANSING FACIAL

1. Cleanse as usual.

2. Use a sauna for five to seven minutes.

3. Wash with scrubbing grains.

4. Rinse with cool water.

5. Apply a gel mask if your skin feels dry or flaky. Use a clay mask if your skin feels irritated, oily, or dirty.

6. Rinse off mask.

7. Apply an astringent if you plan to go out; apply a face lotion if you are going to sleep.

LOW-COST HOMEMADE PREPARATIONS FOR NORMAL SKIN

TONING LOTION FOR NORMAL SKIN
8 ounces witch hazel
½ teaspoon alum
Mix together in bottle. Cover. Keep in refrigerator.

CLAY MASK FOR NORMAL SKIN
1 tablespoon Fuller's earth
1 tablespoon water
1 drop extract of mint
1 pinch alum
Mix everything together to form a paste. Spread on face. Let dry and remain fifteen to twenty minutes. Wash off with cool water.

STIMULATING EGG MASK FOR NORMAL SKIN
1 whole egg, beaten lightly
1 teaspoon honey
¼ teaspoon fresh baker's yeast
Mix all ingredients. Spread on face. Let remain for fifteen or twenty minutes. Wash off with cool water.

. . .

Dry Skin

There are probably more products and treatments available and more attention paid to dry skin than any other type of beauty problem. It would *seem* that just about everyone has dry skin. In reality, this is just not true. True dry skin is fairly rare in girls under twenty-five, and many cases of dry skin in the twenty to thirty age group reflect normal skin that has not been properly cared for. It is a very real problem, however, for women over thirty and must be carefully understood to be controlled and to prevent permanent damage to the skin.

Part of the preoccupation with dry skin comes from the belief that dry skin causes wrinkles, and if you could prevent dry skin, wrinkles would not appear. Unfortunately, this has now been shown to be wrong. While wrinkles do seem to accompany dry skin, the two conditions arise from unrelated changes in the body due to aging. Dry skin is so unrelated to wrinkles that one could always wear a layer of cream on the face and still wind up with lines and wrinkles. The skin would be soft, but wrinkled. In Chapter 5—which deals with the problem of aging skin—the causes of wrinkles, lines, and baggy skin are discussed in detail, as well as ways to prevent and care for these skin problems.

Another cause of the overemphasis on dry skin is the image, heavily promoted by cosmetic ads, that dry skin is somehow chic and upper class, while oily skin is coarse and lower class. In this situation, admitting you have oily skin is tantamount to admitting that you are crude and common.

What Causes Dry Skin

The direct cause of dry skin is the loss of too much water, by evaporation from the cells of the skin—not a lack of oil. When the cellular water level falls too low, the cells of the epidermis break apart and are rapidly shed from the skin's surface. The flakes found on dry skin are actually the loose dehydrated cells.

The natural oils produced by the body's oil glands act as a protective film over the skin. This film prevents excessive evaporation of water from the cells of the skin. But when the water level of the skin itself is low, all the commercial greases, oils, and creams in the world cannot by themselves make the skin moist and supple again. The key to caring for dry skin lies in the careful management of its moisture content, or water level.

The water level of the millions of skin cells is controlled by three factors: outside atmosphere, water-attracting compounds, and hormone balance.

OUTSIDE ATMOSPHERE: If the weather is dry, cold, or windy, the cellular water will evaporate quickly from the skin, leaving it flaky and chapped. If, as in England, the prevailing atmosphere is rainy and misty, the skin will benefit from the constant moisture. Many skin experts believe that the beautiful complexions distinguishing so many English girls are due in part to their country's foggy weather.

WATER-ATTRACTING COMPOUNDS: The skin is thought to contain a group of inborn water-attracting compounds located primarily at the barrier level of the epidermis. These natural moisturizing factors (N.M.F.'s) encourage the skin to hold water. Several of the N.M.F. compounds have been isolated from epidermal tissue. These have been synthesized by chemists and are now commercially available.

Other substances have been created that act like natural N.M.F.'s. These and the synthetic N.M.F.'s are the foundation of the moisturizing creams widely available today. Some compounds have a greater ability to attract and hold water than others and are thus better for any skin. Shopping hints for the best moisturizers are given on page 16.

It is significant to note that, as a woman or man grows older, it is thought that the amount of natural N.M.F.'s in their skin tissues decreases; this is one of the reasons why every woman's skin gets dryer as she grows older.

HORMONE BALANCE: The levels of estrogen and progesterone, the female hormones, have two effects on the condition of women's skins:

1. The hormones themselves are water-attracting substances, which puts them in the N.M.F. category. This is how hormone creams work. Spread on the skin, they attract water and give the skin the appearance of fullness and softness.

2. The level of female hormones in the body helps determine the extent of the activity of the oil glands. If their level drops (as happens during menopause), the resulting loss of the protective oil film increases the rate of skin cellular-water evaporation, which causes dry skin.

The hormones in skin creams, however, do not stimulate the oil glands. Only hormone replacement therapy, based on the same or very similar hormones to those found in birth control pills, can increase or alter a woman's internal hormonal levels. Unfortunately, hormone replacement therapy does not seem to help dry skin.

Therefore, on the basis of what is presently known about the causes of dry skin, a rational program of dry-skin care would include: (a) gentle but thorough cleansing; (b) replenishing the skin with water and N.M.F.'s; and (c) application of a protective covering of oil to prevent the excess evaporation of cellular water.

The Care of Dry Skin

CLEANSING: Soap and water have long been banned for dry-skin care. Soap dissolves the layer of surface oil on the skin, leaving the skin without a protective film against excess evaporation of cellular water. Soap also strips off the top layer of loose cells found on dry and normal skins alike. On dry skins, however, these dead skin cells are sloughed off all too readily by themselves.

A plain cream cleanser like cold cream or solidified mineral oil does not remove too much oil and water from the skin; however, it also does not do a good job of cleansing—it leaves a sticky, greasy film on the skin that discolors makeup and makes the complexion look dull and muddy. If a soap or after-cleansing freshener is used to remove the sticky film, the skin will lose too much oil and water, and will become drier.

The most heavily promoted kind of *cleansing cream* is basically a mixture of soap, oil, and wax. It is not good for any type of skin and is particularly bad for dry skin. This product, which is rubbed into the skin and then tissued off, leaves a film containing soap, which draws water out of the skin and dissolves any surface oil present. The lack of water makes the skin very dry. Regardless of whatever other ingredients they contain—even perfectly good moisturizers—these cleansers will not help dry skin. The purpose of a cleanser is to take off the dirt, dead cells, and stale oil from the surface of the skin—not to remain on and condition the skin.

Dry skin, nevertheless, must still be thoroughly cleaned of its dry flaky cells, stale perspiration, and surface dirt. It needs a thorough cleanser that will remove all these things, yet not strip off all the oil and take out too much water. The answer is the *washable cream* (see page 15). This product is rubbed onto the skin, like a cream, and rinsed off thoroughly with water. It does not remove nearly as much oil as soap; it leaves a nongreasy film on the face that inhibits evaporation of water; and, finally, it does not discolor makeup.

It is never necessary, or even helpful, to spend extra money on washable creams with exotic special ingredients such as shark oil, royal jelly, sea salts, honey, or extracts of herbs and flowers. Even if they were of any value, and most of them are not, a cleansing cream is on the skin for too short a time for these generally expensive ingredients to have any effect at all.

SPECIAL CLEANSING: Dry skin gets a lot of buildup of dead cells on its surface. This layer of cells gives the skin a dull, patchy color. To remove this layer, dry skin should be treated once a month with *scrubbing grains* formulated in an oil base (the usual type of scrubbing cleanser used for other types of skin is too harsh and drying for dry skin). An example of this type of product is SWEDISH FORMULA PURIFIED CLEANSING GRAINS by Max Factor. Good homemade versions can also be made quite easily at much less cost. See the recipes on pages 43–4, following the "Program of Care for Dry Skin."

OIL-BALANCE CONTROL: Since dry skin lacks water, it needs the help of a cream (or lotion) that will shield the skin against excessive water evaporation.

Day creams. A good product should have: (a) a high water content to feed water to the skin's cells; (b) many N.M.F.'s to help the skin retain the water; and (c) an oil that is as close to natural sebum as possible to prevent the excess evaporation of water from the skin.

Because a day cream is worn under makeup, it also must be nongreasy.

Most creams are made with water; the thinner the cream,

the greater the amount of water it contains. It is easier for N.M.F.'s, hormones, and vitamins to help the skin in a thinner cream. For these reasons, a thin, lotion-like cream is better for dry skin than a thick one.

Natural moisturizing factors are not always easy to identify from a product's label. Merely because a cream claims to be a moisturizer does not mean that it contains an N.M.F. Three synthesized moisturizers are Lantrol®, Amerlate®, and Aqualizer®. Look for these ingredients on the label before you buy. If the ingredients are not yet listed on the label (it is not mandatory until March 1975), write to the manufacturer for the list of ingredients in his moisturizers. One product which contains Aqualizer® is SECOND DEBUT.

One way to be sure that a cream contains an N.M.F.-like substance (i.e., one that helps the skin hold water) is to buy one that contains estrogen or progesterone. These hormones are thought to act like N.M.F.'s and must be included on the label under current F.D.A. regulations.

Almost every cosmetic manufacturer puts out a hormone cream, and the price range can vary from two dollars per ounce to ten dollars per ounce. The F.D.A. also regulates the amount of hormone allowed in a cream, and most manufacturers use the maximum permitted amount, which is ten thousand units/ounce. The price differential rarely reflects the amount of estrogen units in a cream.

Silicones also encourage the skin to hold water and are thus a valuable addition to a cream for dry skin. Although the F.D.A. does not require the listing of silicone on the label, most manufacturers will mention its presence in a product. They feel it is a good selling point and they are right.

Cosmetic companies frequently promote their day creams (moisturizers or moisturizing creams) on the basis of the various types of oil they contain. As discussed in Chapters 1 and 2, there is very little difference between the values of the assorted oils. Most claims for special properties are highly dubious.

Other additives and substances found in moisturizing creams are discussed in the glossary. Some have value, and others are worthless. Check the glossary before buying a new product to be certain that its ingredients are truly good for your skin.

Night creams. The same cream used during the day under makeup can be used alone at night. A night cream should do the same job as your day cream: retain moisture in your skin. Creams specifically labeled for night use are often greasier than day creams, since there is no problem with makeup discoloration. The additional oils can somewhat increase the protective coating properties of the cream and help the skin to hold more water. If money is tight, however, a day cream can easily double as a night cream.

Eye and throat creams do not provide better care of dry skin than does a good facial moisturizing lotion. These special areas of the face have no unique needs that can be met only by a special cream. It is a waste of money to buy them in addition to your basic moisturizer or night cream.

TONING: The dull, rough appearance of dry skin will be alleviated a great deal by the toning effects of: astringents, face masks, and facial saunas.

Astringents. Women with dry skin should be very wary of commercial astringents—even if they are advertised as suitable for dry skin. In order to give a fresh, cool feeling to the skin, all such products usually contain a rapidly drying substance such as alcohol, which will leach water out of the already water-poor dry skin. The astringents that claim to contain no alcohol usually contain another chemical with the same drying properties as alcohol. The same holds true for astringent-like products, such as pore lotions, skin fresheners, skin tonics, and so forth.

Dry skin can, nonetheless, derive a great deal of benefit from an astringent. The aluminum salts in such a product will make pores seem smaller and generally make the skin seem firmer. Until all the cosmetic companies have listed their formulas on the products (by 1975), it is best to make your own dry-skin astringent from water and aluminum salts.

DRY-SKIN ASTRINGENT
1 cup distilled water (available in drugstores)
½ teaspoon alum
   (the most easily available aluminum salt)
Shake well and store in the refrigerator.

This homemade astringent must be refrigerated for two very important reasons. First of all, cold itself is an astringent, so refrigeration will improve the mixture's pore-shrinking ability. At the same time, the low temperature will prevent the growth of bacteria, a real problem, since this astringent does not contain preservatives. Be sure to label and date the jar carefully so that no one will drink it by mistake. While it is not poison, it is not a good idea to drink it. At the end of three months, throw out what remains, and make a new batch.

Face masks. Face masks can help dry skin in several ways. Any mask spread over the surface of the face forms a watertight shield. This shield, which usually remains on the skin for about thirty minutes, allows the tissues to build up a rich supply of water. The tightening action of the mask stimulates the skin's circulation. Finally, when the mask is removed many of the loose flaky cells are pulled off, leaving the skin's surface smooth and soft.

Gel-type masks are the best for dry skin. They help the skin build up a good supply of water and remove the dry scaly cells on the surface of the skin. Two examples of the gel mask for dry skin include Shiseido's FACIAL PACK (EXTRA RICH), and Revlon's MOISTURIZING HONEY MASQUE.

As mentioned earlier, estrogens, N.M.F.'s, and silicones present in a mask help the skin retain water. Other additives to masks may be useless; check the Glossary.

Clay masks, while they do the same things as gel masks, also absorb the surface oil of the skin. This makes them wonderful for oily and acne-troubled skin, but less than satisfactory for dry skin.

Facial saunas. These are a vital part of dry-skin care. An inexpensive commercial home sauna device, or the more economical sauna improvised with a pot of water and a towel, provides three very important functions in the care of dry skin: (a) a sauna delivers a wonderful moist atmosphere to cover the skin like a mist; (b) a sauna provides steam at a safe low temperature that cleans the pores by dissolving the stale oil on the skin; (c) the heat of the sauna's moist steam gently stimulates oil gland production in the skin.

Makeup and Dry Skin

Women with dry skin should use cream and oil-based makeup exclusively. Foundations that are light but rich in oil are best for dry skin. Smoothed over a day cream, they provide another film of oil to slow down the evaporation of water from the skin. On the other hand, heavy oily foundations usually contain soaps or other drying emulsifiers to make them thicker.

Women with dry skin should never use powder because it soaks up oil and water, the two essential skin moisturizers. Another product to avoid is any form of pancake makeup. These are compounded principally of soap and clay—and are drying to all but the oiliest skins.

Women with dry skin should use creamy eye makeup, lipsticks, and blushers. Beware of frosted cosmetics, however; the ingredients that give the skin a frosted look or a pearly sheen can also prove to be drying agents. The sheen is produced by tiny amounts of minerals, which soak up water and natural oils. Although these cosmetics can make a dry skin appear fresh and smooth at first, if the skin seems dryer several hours after applying a frosted makeup, it should not be used again.

Today, a clear, glossy look is very popular. Cosmetics that help produce this look contain a high proportion of gels. When used as a foundation, however, they might not provide the same complete protection against excess evaporation of natural skin moisture that is available in a richer, oilier foundation.

Foundations for dry skin should be tested on the inside of the forearm. If they disappear into the skin quickly, leaving only a faint trace of color, leave them on the cosmetics counter and keep looking. You need a foundation that will make a thicker covering for the skin.

A PROGRAM OF CARE FOR DRY SKIN

NIGHT

1. Clean the face with washable cleanser according to the package directions. Rinse very well, splashing about twenty handfuls of warm water on the face. Then dry the face in the air, keeping out of drafts.

2. Pat moisturizer into the skin.

3. Try to get at least eight hours of sleep. Since the skin cells are thought to do most of their growing when the body is at rest, insufficient sleep might not give the skin an opportunity to replenish itself.

DAY CARE

1. Cleanse your face as you did for night care.
2. Apply astringent with a fresh ball of cotton.
3. Let your face dry.
4. Apply a moisturizer.
5. Now apply your makeup.

WEEKLY FACIAL

1. Cleanse the face lightly with a washable cream and rinse well.
2. Steam the face over a sauna for five minutes.
3. Rinse off with cool water.
4. Rub in a cream-based scrubbing grain around your chin, nose, cheeks, and forehead. Rinse off with tepid water.
5. Apply the gel face mask. Let it dry.
6. If you have the time, lie down on your bed with your head hanging back over the edge of the bed. Stay in this position for ten minutes! This will bring the blood to the head and give your skin a rosy glow.
7. Rinse off the mask.
8. Apply an astringent.
9. Apply a moisturizer lotion.
10. Now apply makeup as desired.

LOW-COST HOMEMADE PREPARATIONS FOR DRY SKIN

DRY-SKIN CLEANSER I

1 teaspoon standard scrubbing cleanser like BRASIVOL or PERNOX
2 tablespoons washable cleanser
Combine the two ingredients. Rub mixture gently all over face. Rinse off thoroughly with cool water. Use once a week.

DRY-SKIN ASTRINGENT I
1 cup distilled water
½ teaspoon alum
   (the most easily available aluminum salt)
Shake well and store in the refrigerator.

DRY-SKIN ASTRINGENT II
8 ounces distilled water
½ teaspoon alum
1 drop extract of mint
Mix together. Store in covered container in refrigerator.

DRY-SKIN CLEANSER II
1 teaspoon washable cleanser
½ teaspoon cornmeal
Mix together. Rub mixture gently all over face. Rinse off
thoroughly with cool water. Use once a week.

DRY-SKIN MASK I
1 egg yolk
1 pinch of alum
1 tablespoon Fuller's earth
1 teaspoon honey
Mix together into a paste. Spread on face.

DRY-SKIN MASK II
1 tablespoon mayonnaise
1 teaspoon Fuller's earth
1 drop extract of mint
1 pinch alum
Mix into a paste. Spread on face. Leave on for twenty minutes. Rinse off with cool water.

Oily Skin

Almost everyone has oily skin during adolescence. It is so
oily that the face is almost always shiny and is prone to acne break-

outs. Dandruff is also common; the hair is greasy and needs frequent washings. By the time age twenty rolls around, this huge outpouring of oil usually slows down, and skin and hair problems disappear.

In many people, however, the oil production does not slow down enough. Although not as oily as before, the face is still prone to acne problems, the hair continues to be greasy, and the skin retains its annoying oily sheen. Dandruff also persists. However, adult oily skin is different from the teenaged version, and, more important, it must be treated differently.

What Causes Oily Skin

The oil glands are very sensitive organs. They react to the balance of hormones in the body, to irritating substances in food, and to changes in the air and the weather. Oil glands can even be affected by your genetic background. Oily skin can be caused by all or any combination of these factors.

HORMONES: In normal skin, some of the hormones secreted by the adrenal glands (androgens) and the hormones secreted by the ovaries (estrogens) are in a fixed ratio in the blood depending upon the age, sex, and state of health of a person. When this ratio becomes disturbed by a variation in either androgen or estrogen levels, it signals the oil glands to produce more oil. A slight difference in hormone levels may not be enough to disturb the rest of the body, but for the sensitive oil glands the slightest shift is enough to start them overproducing.

DIET: There is even less certainty about the role diet plays with oily skin than there is about diet and acne. While most people firmly believe that certain foods (e.g., chocolate, fats, citrus fruits, seafood, and hot spices) make the skin oilier, there is no concrete proof for this idea. It might very well be that some people's skins do become oilier after eating these foods, but there are probably other factors that originally made their skin oily. At most, certain foods may make an already oily skin somewhat oilier, but they are never the sole reason for this type of skin.

While it probably doesn't hurt to avoid these foods, overreliance on diet can lead one to ignore the more important causes and treatments for oily skin.

ENVIRONMENT: Oily skin is sensitive to changes in the weather. A hot, humid climate stimulates secretion from the oil glands. It is felt that heavily polluted air contains chemicals that can irritate the oil glands, making them produce excess oil. People with oily skin who live in cities or in hot damp climates must take extra care of their skin.

GENETICS: Certain ethnic groups seem to be more prone to oily skin than others. Mediterranean peoples with olive skin and dark hair are thought to have more (or perhaps more active) oil glands than do the fair, light-skinned people of Scandinavian or Scottish descent, and thus are more troubled with the problems of oily skin.

The Care of Oily Skin

Oily skin is probably the easiest skin problem to control successfully. There is no tissue damage as with dry skin or acne; oily skin is basically healthy skin. The oil provides an excellent shield against water evaporation; in addition, oily skin shows the signs of aging less than do other types of skin.

Oily skin needs thorough cleansing, a mild drying agent, and nongreasy makeup. Oily skin never *needs* any creams or moisturizers; it produces more than enough oils naturally, and any additional creams will change oily skin into acned skin. One of the leading causes of acne in those adults is the needless use of cleansing creams, lubricants, night oils, and moisturizers (these being primarily emulsions of *oil* and water).

Certainly everyone's skin requires moisture to keep it from becoming dry, rough, and flaky. The skin loses its moisture through evaporation from the skin's surface, but this evaporation occurs only if the skin lacks a natural protective coat of oil. Oily skin hardly lacks oil. A moisturizer will glue the layer of dead cells more tightly together, obstructing pore openings, and making the face greasy.

Never use any cream, lotion, or moisturizer on your face if you have oily skin.

CLEANSING:

Soaps. You need a soap that is stronger than regular soap, but not as strong as those soaps used for acne. Look for a soap with a low concentration of sulfur (2 to 3 percent), and/or resorcinol (1 to 2 percent), as well as a disinfectant like alcohol or acetone. A good example of such a soap is ACNE AID SOAP by Stiefel. Check your labels very carefully. Many highly touted soaps for oily skin contain only alcohol. Alcohol will check the growth of bacteria but it does not have the drying power of sulfur, resorcinol, or scrubbing grains.

Scrubbing grains. These are soaps containing little grains that act as an abrasive on the skin. One of the great problems of oily skin is that the oil causes the top layer of dead skin cells to clump together, making them much harder to remove. It is this top layer that makes the skin look thick and muddy. The scrubbing grains scrape off the top layer of cells, making the skin look smoother and clearer. Two examples of this product are PERNOX and BRASIVOL.

OIL-BALANCE CONTROL:

Drying lotions. You will want a mild drying cream with enough sulfur, resorcinol, and salicylic acid to discourage the production of oil by the oil glands and, at the same time, a lotion that can remove the layer of dead dry skin cells. An example of this type of product is pHISOAC by Winthrop or FOSTRIL by Westwood Pharmaceuticals.

TONING:

Astringents. Find an astringent with alcohol, alum, and a balanced pH. The balanced pH is fairly important, because you want to help maintain the acid mantle, which is one of the skin's natural barriers against infection. If you cannot find an astringent with these qualities add one-half teaspoonful of powdered alum (sold in supermarkets) to eight ounces of a plain alcohol-based face tonic or freshener like TEN-O-SIX LOTION by Bonne Bell or PORE LOTION by Almay.

Face masks. Clay-based masks do very good things for oily skin. They absorb excess oil from the top layer of the skin and remove dirt and dead cells. One such mask is 5-MINUTE FACIAL MASK by Almay.

Special additives can increase the value of a clay mask.

Sulfur, resorcinol, and salicylic acid will slow down the activity of the oil glands. At the same time they help strip off the layer of congealed oil and dead cells. Alcohol can increase the drying power of a mask. As usual, watch out for useless ingredients: for example, herbs, as a rule, can do little to help oily skin. The same is true of flower and vegetable extracts, strawberries, cucumbers, and grapefruits. These are good foods in your diet, but are ineffective when added to cosmetics. For further details on individual additives, check the references listed in the Glossary.

Saunas. Facial saunas are vital to the care of oily skin. The moist heat of the sauna melts the oil stuck in the follicles, loosens the top layer of dead cells stuck to the skin's surface, and feeds a nice dose of water to the skin. This water will keep the skin—which is being treated with strong degreasing soaps and drying lotions— from becoming too rough and flaky. It is the water in the skin that keeps it soft and smooth, not the oil.

Makeup and Oily Skin

The best makeup for oily skin is an oil-free cosmetic. Almay, Ar-Ex, and Revlon each have a line of oil-free products. Almay and Ar-Ex are hypo-allergenic in that they contain no perfume or other known major irritant. Be careful; some products advertised as hypoallergenic or medicated contain as much oil as regular cosmetics.

If you want to get regular cosmetics, be sure to avoid the extremely greasy products. Pancake makeup, cream foundation, creamy rouge, and super-thick lipsticks all contain huge amounts of oil. Use liquid foundation, dry brush-on rouge and eye shadow, and a light lipstick.

A PROGRAM OF CARE FOR OILY SKIN

NIGHT

1. Wash with soap: Wet your hands and face, and work up a good lather. Rub this lather on the face all the way up to your hair line and down under the chin. Pay special attention to the forehead, nose, and chin areas. If the lather dries up, add more soap and water. Rinse off well with about six handfuls of lukewarm water. If you use a lot of eye makeup,

remove it with eye-makeup remover pads or a bit of mineral oil or cold cream before washing the rest of the face. Be certain to remove all traces of the oil and take care not to get the oil on the other parts of the face.

2. With a clean cotton ball, put on an astringent. This should be done faithfully every night. Let it dry.

3. Rub drying lotion all over the face.

DAY

1. Wash as for the night.

2. Use an astringent as for night.

3. For the first weeks of this program use a drying lotion during the day, alone or under makeup. Then use it only at night. Makeup can be applied directly to the freshly washed face. Do not use powder. Oily skin will just discolor and cake it; in addition, powder will ultimately clog your pores. Once you have made up your face, do not add more makeup during the day—even if your face is shiny—until you've cleaned your face. A prepackaged towelette specially made for oily skin (e.g., SEBA-NIL by Texas Pharmacal Co.) is a handy touchup; then reapply your makeup. This is not a substitute for soap and water cleaning, which is preferable, if at all possible.

WEEKLY DEEP-CLEANSING

1. Wash face thoroughly with soap. Rinse.

2. Steam for ten minutes with sauna.

3. Scrub with cleansing grains.

4. Rinse thoroughly with cool water.

5. Put on clay mask and let dry.

6. Rinse off, pat with an astringent.

7. Rub on drying lotion.

LOW-COST HOMEMADE PREPARATIONS FOR OILY SKIN

OILY-SKIN ASTRINGENT

4 ounces alcohol

4 ounces distilled water
½ teaspoon alum
Mix together. Keep covered in refrigerator.

OILY-SKIN CLAY MASK

2 tablespoons alcohol
1 tablespoon Fuller's earth
Mix to a paste and apply to face.

4 / Acne: The Most Common Skin Problem

Acne is the most common and troublesome skin problem. It is found in 80 percent of all teenagers and many adults as well. It consists of blackheads, greasy skin, pimples, large pores, and in severe cases, scarring and cyst-like eruptions. Acne is primarily caused by overactive oil glands, which are influenced by the body's hormonal changes, diet, and extremely warm weather, as well as by genetic factors.

The Causes of Acne

Hormones

The adrenal glands secrete androgens as well as other non-sex-related hormones; in women, the ovaries secrete estrogens as well as other female sex hormones, and in men, androgens (male sex hormones) are secreted by the testes as well as the adrenal glands. In women, the sole source of androgens is the adrenal glands.

These hormones are produced in ratios to one another depending on age, sex, and other natural factors. That is to say, for a given individual there exists a ratio in which these hormones are normally present. During puberty, the adrenal glands produce large quantities of androgen—sometimes as much as three to four times the prepuberty amount. This production is not abnormal, since these hormones are needed to produce the growth of bones as well as the proper maturation of sexual characteristics. It is unfortunate that the increase of these hormones also stimulates the oil glands to produce too much oil. The oil accumulates in the follicle, giving rise to the all too familiar signs of acne: blackheads, whiteheads, pimples, and cysts.

A blackhead, or open comedone in medical terms, is a solid plug of oil that is lodged in the neck of the follicle (see Diagram 4A). Many doctors feel that its dark color is due to a chemical change that results from exposure to the air. Left alone, the blackhead will remain unchanged. The oil glands attached to the blackhead-clogged follicle shrink somewhat in size and decrease oil production. A pimple will not form from a blackhead, unless it is disturbed by picking or improper extraction. Most pimples arise from the whitehead.

The whitehead, or closed comedone, begins when excess oil produced by overstimulated oil glands gets clogged up in a follicle (see Diagram 4B). The increased amounts of oil irritate the cells of the follicle wall, making them fall off more rapidly into the follicle. When these extra cells accumulate over the opening of the

Diagram 4.

B. WHITEHEAD

A. BLACKHEAD

The blackhead, or open comedone, is a small plug of darkened sebum that has lodged at the neck of the follicle.

Blackhead

Note that there is no oil in the other parts of the follicle.

The whitehead, or closed comedone, is caused by an accumulation of dead skin cells and sebum in the follicle; a growth of skin cells covers the opening, making it impossible for this matter to move out of the pore.

Skin has grown over the opening of the pore.

Oil has backed up in the follicle.

D. CYST

C. PIMPLE

A pimple begins when the follicle walls start to leak oil and dead cells into the surrounding dermis.

If the follicle leaks a great deal of matter deep into the dermis, a wall will sometimes form around the leaked oil-cell mixture, thus causing a painful cyst.

—Leak

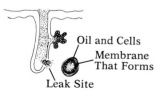

Oil and Cells
Membrane
That Forms
Leak Site

follicle they seal up all the cells and oil inside. The whitehead is seen on the surface of the skin as a slightly raised white lump. At this point (see Diagram 4C) the bacteria that normally live in the oil follicle begin to change the chemistry of the oil, forming free fatty acids. The fatty acids seem to stimulate both the oil glands to produce more oil and the cells of the follicle to increase and fall off, filling the follicle even more. This additional material causes the follicle to swell. The comedone is about to become a pimple.

The pimple begins when the follicle, weakened by its increased load of oil, cells, and bacteria, develops a break and leaks some of its contents into the dermis, the skin's lower layer (see Diagram 4C). The oil-cells-bacteria mixture is very irritating to the dermis and causes an inflammatory condition. White blood cells now rush to "help" the inflamed area, causing the creation of pus. The inflammation appears on the skin as a raised, red, round area. If the follicle breaks near the surface of the skin, the pimple is small, short-lived, and does not cause any damage to the skin. When the follicle breaks deep in the dermis, the pimple is far more severe. It is larger, frequently warm, painful, and filled with pus. Such pimples take one to two weeks to heal and can leave deeply red or purple areas on the skin that last for months.

A cyst arises when the follicle break occurs quite deep in the dermis and a large amount of oil is leaked; a wall forms around the leaked material (see Diagram 4D). This structure appears as a large, raised, hard, painful lump under the skin's surface. The cyst lasts much longer than even a very severe pimple. In fact, very few cysts ever go away without medical treatment. Cysts destroy a good deal of skin and frequently leave permanent scars.

Not everyone has the same amount of acne. There are, in fact, four grades of acne problems:

Grade 1. This consists only of blackheads and whiteheads on the face. There are few or no pimples.

Grade 2. The skin is noticeably oily. There are whiteheads, blackheads, and pimples located primarily on the face, but in some cases these can appear on the back and chest as well. This is the most common form of adolescent acne. It does not cause scarring.

Grade 3. The skin is extremely oily. There are many whiteheads, blackheads, large pus-filled pimples, and deep hard lumps that are cysts. Grade 3 acne can cover the face, neck, shoulders, and upper back. It frequently causes scarring.

Grade 4. The skin is excessively oily; there are many large cysts overlapping one another, forming raised, thickened areas on the skin. The resulting scars form cord-like ridges on the skin's surface.

Although the root of all acne problems is the increased amount of oil in the follicles primarily as a result of hormonal changes, stress, diet, extremely warm weather, and heredity also play a role.

Stress

Many people blame tension or emotional problems for all their acne. While it is true that stress can make an existing acne condition somewhat worse, stress alone cannot create a case of acne on normal skin, nor can it change a mild case into an extremely severe one. We all live under varying degrees of stress beyond our control, and it is far more productive to concentrate on causes of acne that we can cope with, like decreasing the amount of surface oil and taking off the cells that are clogging the pores.

Diet

Many different foods have been blamed for acne. While the exact chemistry in each case is different, all these foods are thought to provoke acne by stimulating the oil glands in some way to over-produce oil. However, the role of diet in acne is now felt to have been vastly overrated. There is no definite scientific evidence that diet is an important cause of acne and, in fact, some experiments have shown that such foods as chocolates and fats do *not* cause or worsen acne conditions. But until the final word is in, many dermatologists still suggest that acne patients stop eating or at least severely limit their intake of sodas, chocolate, fried foods, citrus fruits, tomatoes, and shellfish.

While there is no harm in avoiding these foods, an overemphasis on diet has frequently led people to ignore the more fundamental causes of acne, such as excess oil and clogged pores. In avoiding pizzas and french fries, they feel they don't need effective acne soaps and lotions. Without this basic skin care acne can never improve, even with the most perfect anti-acne diet.

Hot Weather

High temperatures and high humidity can increase oil gland production. While sunbathing can cause an improvement in acne, mostly because the skin peels after sunburn, some people find their acne is made worse by the sun.

Genetic Factors

Acne is not an inherited trait like blue eyes or curly hair. However, there is usually a history of acne in the family of a person with acne. If one or both of your parents had acne, the chances are good that you will have it too. Your acne will probably also be of the same severity and resolve itself at about the same age.

The Care of Adolescent Acne

The control of adolescent acne should be directed at lessening the amount of oil the skin produces. Changing the hormone balance with estrogen pills to discourage the oil glands would seem to be the simplest way to slow down oil production. However, the hormone imbalance that causes acne in adolescents is part of the maturation process. Tampering with hormones at this time leads to serious health problems. However, as we shall see in the next chapter, estrogen therapy is sometimes used for acne problems in women past puberty.

The care of adolescent acne begins with a proper cleansing and drying program that will remove excess oil and the accumulation of dead cells that are blocking the follicles.

Cleansing

Cleansing begins with special anti-acne soaps containing chemicals that:
1. Dissolve oil.
2. Break down dead cells.
3. Slow down oil-gland activity.

In order to meet these special requirements soaps for acne contain specific chemicals. Two or more of these chemicals should always be present in an acne soap; these are sulfur, alcohol, resorcinol, and salicylic acid.

SULFUR: This decreases the activity of the oil glands and at the same time causes some of the skin's dead cells to peel off.

ALCOHOL: This acts as a disinfectant.

RESORCINOL AND SALICYLIC ACID: These are excellent peeling agents. They remove the top layer of dead cells that plugs up the pores.

All these chemicals are required by present F.D.A. law to be listed on the label of any cosmetic product in which they are found. If there are no such ingredients listed, the soap will not do a good job on acned skin.

Plain soaps alone will, to some extent, dissolve oils and remove dead tissue, but soaps containing anti-acne chemicals will do a more thorough job. Two such soaps are FOSTEX by Westwood Pharmaceuticals and SASTID SOAP by Stiefel. However, even after you have washed with a good anti-acne soap, oil plugs can still remain wedged within the follicle; the oil becomes hardened and sticks to the walls of the follicles. There is absolutely no substance available that reaches down into plugged pores and cleans them out. Don't believe any ad that claims this feat for its product.

The best way to deep-clean the pores yourself is to use *hot packs*; simply soak a washcloth in very hot water, and apply it to all parts of the face, with the exception of the eyes and mouth. The moist heat of the hot pack will melt the hardened oil; it will also expand your pores and thus encourage them to give up their oils naturally.

After steaming in this manner, a thorough washing with a good anti-acne soap will remove any of the oil that has seeped out of the dilated pores. In addition, washing will remove the top layer of tissue that was loosened by steaming.

Acne-troubled skin will also derive great benefit from soaps containing scrubbing grains. These rub off the dead skin clogging the pores and give the follicles a chance to rid themselves of excess oil. This type of soap also removes blackheads and makes the skin seem brighter and fresher. Be sure to choose this soap in a nonoily form. Two such products are BRASIVOL and PERNOX.

Once the skin has been cleansed of its oil and dead skin, an acne lotion containing at least two or more of the same chemicals found in a good acne soap (sulfur, resorcinol, salicylic acid, and alcohol) can discourage the oil from building up again. Acne lotions should be worn day and night to keep oil production at a minimum and the skin free from all cell buildup. Some of these products are designed to look like makeup foundations and hide existing blemishes while they work to prevent further breakouts. Four such products are ACNE-DOME (Dome), pHISOAC CREAM (Winthrop), ACNOMEL (Smith, Kline & French), and FOSTRIL (Westwood).

Be very wary of the so-called medicated foundations put out by several cosmetic companies. As with so many cosmetic terms, there is no legal definition of what medicated means, and at present it means anything the manufacturer wishes. Sometimes these products contain alcohol, which is a good disinfectant, but this is not enough to really help acned skin.

Other "medicated" foundations are much less oily than regular foundations. Again, this is good, but not as beneficial as a lotion containing active anti-acne chemicals.

Always read the label of a medicated foundation. If it does not contain at least two of the effective anti-acne chemicals, do not buy it.

Toning

Acne-troubled skin thrives on good toning procedures. As always, toning begins with an astringent.

ASTRINGENTS: An astringent should disinfect, make pores seem smaller, dissolve any remaining oils, and help maintain the acid balance of the skin.

Look for a product containing alcohol and/or sulfur, resorcinol, or salicylic acid. Some products contain lime or lemon extract, which gives the astringent an acid pH. This is excellent for acned skin. Two such products are PROPA pH and TEN-O-SIX LOTION (Bonne Bell).

· · ·

FACE MASKS: Acned skin derives great benefit from face masks based on clay. The clay absorbs surface oil and picks up loose dead skin cells. As the clay tightens, it stimulates the circulation of the blood. When the clay mask is removed it takes the loose dead skin cells with it.

The basis for the activity of a good mask is the clay, but certain additives can increase the value of these masks for acne control. The same four chemicals found in acne soaps and lotions (sulfur, resorcinol, salicylic acid, and alcohol) will perform their anti-acne functions in a clay mask. An example of this type of mask is 5-MINUTE FACIAL MASK by Almay.

Check the Glossary for information about other additives used in anti-acne masks, soaps, and lotions.

Makeup

Makeup should be as oil-free as possible; a dry rouge or blush and eyeshadow should be used, and oily, super-rich lipstick should be avoided.

A PROGRAM OF CARE FOR ACNE-TROUBLED SKIN

DAY

1. Wash with special acne soap, making sure you scrub the top of the forehead, the nose, the chin, around the lips, and the cheeks as well.

2. Rinse well with water.

3. Use scrubbing-grain soap according to the package directions.

4. Apply an astringent with a small cotton ball—using a fresh one each time.

5. Wait for the astringent to dry.

6. With your fingers apply an acne lotion, spreading it over the whole face, not just dabbing it in spots where the face is broken out. This will prevent new eruptions and heal old ones as well.

. . .

NIGHT

1. Wash with acne soap as you did in the morning.

2. Fill up the bottom of the sink with very hot water. Soak two washcloths in this water. Protecting your hands with rubber gloves, take one out, wring it, and apply it to your face. The face can take the hot water better than your hands. When this cloth cools, put it back into the hot water, and then repeat using the other washcloth. Do this ten to fifteen minutes every night.

3. With a cotton ball, pat on an astringent and let it dry.

4. With your fingers smooth on acne lotion. Put it on thickly.

TWICE-WEEKLY DEEP-CLEANSING

Twice a week instead of your usual nightly care the following should be done to treat your acne thoroughly (more frequent use of this program may lead to irritation of the skin).

1. Wash with acne soap.

2. Wash with scrubbing grains.

3. Apply hot towels for five minutes.

4. Rinse your face in cool (not cold) water. Cold water will be too much of a shock for the skin and may break some blood vessels.

5. Apply a clay mask and leave it on for thirty minutes.

6. Wash off the mask with cool water; dry your face.

7. Apply an astringent.

8. Apply an acne lotion.

LOW-COST HOMEMADE PREPARATIONS FOR ACNE-TROUBLED SKIN

ACNE ASTRINGENT

½ cup witch hazel
½ cup alcohol
½ teaspoon alum
1 drop extract of mint
Mix together and store in screw-top bottle in refrigerator.

. . .

ACNE TREATMENT MASK
2 teaspoons acne cream or lotion
2 teaspoons Fuller's earth
Mix into paste. Let remain for thirty minutes.

ACNE CLAY MASK
2 tablespoons calamine lotion
1 tablespoon Fuller's earth
Mix together to paste. Spread on face.

This basic cleansing and drying program will, under normal circumstances, control Grade 1 and 2 acne (which are the degrees of acne that most adolescents have). It is especially effective if started early, right after acne first appears. However, Grade 3 and 4 acne, and sometimes even Grade 2 acne that has gone on for several years, will need the care available only through a dermatologist. The following sections review some of the techniques dermatologists use, as well as what you should and shouldn't expect of them.

Techniques Dermatologists Use

SLUSH BATHS: These consist of a mixture of powdered carbon dioxide, acetone, and powdered sulfur. This mixture is applied with a wad of gauze to the whole face. It is very cold and makes strange spluttering sounds. After a few moments on the skin, the acetone and the carbon dioxide evaporate, leaving a fine deposit of sulfur on the face. This is allowed to remain for twenty minutes; it is then rinsed off and a regular acne lotion is applied. The slush bath treatment causes peeling of the skin's outer layer as well as the smoothing of the skin's surface. It discourages new eruption formation and, at the same time, helps to reduce old acne scars. Obviously this elaborate and potent treatment should be administered only by a qualified dermatologist. Improper use can cause deep burns and severe scarring. This is *not* a do-it-yourself or beauty-shop procedure.

The slush bath used in strong concentrations is one of the best ways of handling large cysts, which are found in Grade 3 and 4 acne. The slush seems to encourage the cysts to open up and release their contents without causing scar tissue.

CORTISONE: Another approach is the injection of cortisone directly into a deep cyst. This drug reduces the inflammation within the cyst and causes it to recede without leaving scar tissue. Cortisone will be mentioned often in this book. It is a hormone that suppresses all kinds of inflammation on the skin and is therefore a useful drug for the control of many skin problems. However, it should never be used without a doctor's supervision. Cortisone, while an extremely effective drug for many skin problems, can have severe side-effects if used for long periods of time.

LANCING: Sometimes a dermatologist decides that a cyst must be lanced (cut open) in order for it to heal. As you remember, the cyst has lost its passage to the skin's surface. With a surgical instrument the dermatologist makes a tiny cut into the top of the cyst. This creates a hole through which the cyst can finally release its contents and, when it does, the skin begins to heal.

Dermatologists also use special medications not available without prescription. They can tailor a night lotion to your complexion needs by adding more sulfur, resorcinol, or alcohol than is available in the nonprescription products. They can also add cortisone to suppress the inflammations and help halt pimple formation.

TETRACYCLINE: Dermatologists also prescribe tetracycline, an antibiotic that has been shown to dramatically improve some cases of acne. Tetracycline reduces the acne by changing the chemical nature of the oil produced by the follicles. You will remember that it is the excess oil in the follicles that causes an increase in the growth of skin cells around the follicle, and that these cells grow over the follicle opening and seal up the oil inside. Scientists now think that the *fatty acids* in the oil are the components that stimulate the increase in cell growth, and that these fatty acids actually stimulate the oil glands to produce more oil. Tetracycline alters the chemistry of the fatty acids so that they no longer stimulate the oil glands to produce more oil or the skin around the follicle to produce more cells. Tetracycline capsules are often given in low doses over a period of months for the care of acne.

VITAMIN A ACID: This, in lotion form, is one of the newer substances found to be effective against acne. It works by stopping the excess growth of cells around the follicles and by vigorously peeling away the layers of cells that clog the pores. At first vitamin A acid seems to make the acne grow worse, but after several weeks of treatment the skin becomes less oily and has fewer blackheads and eruptions. Vitamin A acid is sold only by prescription from a physician, and should never be used except under the supervision of a doctor.

VITAMIN A CAPSULES: These are also used for acne control. When taken in the proper dose this vitamin has the ability to slow the overgrowth of cells around the follicle, diminishing the problems of plugged-up pores, and thus reducing the incidence of pimples.

While vitamin A is a good additional weapon in the fight against acne, excess vitamin A consumption has been shown to produce very serious health problems. The tendency to think that "if one vitamin pill is good then three must be terrific" has led to the complications of excess vitamin A, which include hair loss, stomach disorders, and, in one frightening case in Washington, D.C., brain damage. Let your doctor determine the dose in your individual case.

Research into the causes and control of acne is continuing, and as a result new techniques are tried and old ones discarded. Two methods of acne care that have dropped from the favor of many doctors are X-ray therapy and ultraviolet treatment.

Outmoded Treatments

X-RAY THERAPY: In past years this was used in extremely severe cases of acne. The X-rays slowed down the activity of the oil glands by destroying the highly active cells that make up the sebaceous glands. The theory was that they would secrete much less sebum. This method of treatment, however, has fallen into disrepute in recent years because it has been shown to be relatively ineffective in the long run and, most important, the X-rays are harmful to the skin and have been implicated in the occurrence of skin cancers many years after the initial treatment.

ULTRAVIOLET TREATMENT (uv): For many years such treatment was used for acne patients. It causes various degrees of peeling as a result of cell destruction by its rays. Many dermatologists have either stopped or at least limited the use of uv treatment. To be at all effective it must be given frequently—at least three times weekly for a period of several weeks. This can be very expensive for a patient when each visit costs a minimum of ten to fifteen dollars.

Buying and using an ultraviolet lamp at home is usually discouraged because of the high number of burns associated with self-treatment. Many people fall asleep under the soothing warmth only to find, on awakening, second- and even first-degree burns. Cases of permanently impaired vision have resulted from overexposure to ultraviolet under such circumstances. There are so many other, more effective, safer, and less expensive ways of caring for acne today that it is not necessary to use ultraviolet treatments.

The Treatment of Acne Scars

Many cases of acne leave scarring that remains after the active period of outbreaks is over. These can be quite unattractive and even disfiguring. Fortunately, there are methods that can remove these scars or make them less obvious. There are three different types of scars resulting from acne: "ice pick" scars, saucer-shaped scars, and raised lumpy scars.

"Ice pick" scars look like giant pores. They are called "ice pick" scars because they appear as if made by a thin, sharp instrument. They are caused by an extremely large pimple or a cyst that has totally destroyed the follicle passage and its oil gland. The total destruction of these structures has literally left a hole in the skin where the follicle once was.

Diagram 5.

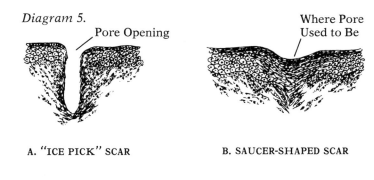

A. "ICE PICK" SCAR   B. SAUCER-SHAPED SCAR

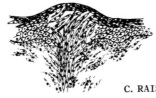

Diagram 5.

C. RAISED LUMPY SCAR

Saucer-shaped scars and raised lumpy scars arise primarily from cysts. The cyst has destroyed the area of skin all the way down through the dermis. The dermis cannot grow back normal skin, only scar tissue. If this scar tissue is below the surface of the skin, the scar will look like a saucer-shaped pit. If there are several large cysts located close to one another and they heal by scarring, the scar tissue rises up and forms the third type of scarring, the raised lumpy scar.

Dermabrasion

"Ice pick" scars and pits are frequently helped by dermabrasion. This technique uses a motor-driven wire brush to remove the epidermis and the very top layers of the dermis. With these top levels of skin planed away, the pits and holes do not look as deep as before. However, the scars and holes go too deep into the dermis to be removed. Any attempt to plane down to the bottom level of the scars would result in disfiguring scar formation, since the dermis cannot regrow normal skin after injury. By planing away the surrounding skin, the acne scars and pits seem shallower and are less noticeable.

Dermabrasion is sometimes used as therapy for active acne. The planing action destroys many oil glands and by taking off the top layers it makes the follicle shorter and thicker. This shape makes it easier for the oil secreted by those oil glands not destroyed by dermabrasion to get out of the follicle.

Cosmetic Surgery

"Ice pick" scars and acne pits can also be helped by face lifting, a technique more commonly used for the removal of lines and wrinkles. In the case of postacne scars the face lift pulls up the skin, smoothing it out and thereby lessening the depth of the acne pits and scars.

The raised lumpy scars do not respond well to dermabrasion. They are sometimes helped by the injection of cortisone directly into the raised scar area.

Some doctors will cut out the scarred raised tissue. This leaves a flat scarred area of the skin, which in certain cases can be successfully treated with dermabrasion.

Because most cases of acne scarring have more than one type of scar, doctors can use several methods to make the skin clear and smooth. Large raised scars can be cut out or alternately injected with cortisone and then the whole face can be treated with dermabrasion. Deep pits that have not been smoothed out by dermabrasion can be built up with minute amounts of *silicone*. However, this technique remains experimental because of questions as to its safety raised by its use in plastic surgery.

Any treatment undertaken for acne scarring should be done only under the supervision of a dermatologist or plastic surgeon. There are many untrained cosmetologists and beauticians who offer dangerous and often useless treatments for acne scars.

Chemical-peeling

The most common procedure the beautician or cosmetologist offers is the *chemical peel*, which uses a caustic substance that burns off the top layers of the skin in an effort to remove acne scars. While this is basically the same principle as dermabrasion, it is much harder to control the depth to which the solution removes the skin. If the chemical goes into the dermis, the skin will grow back only scar tissue. Instead of having a few areas with scars, the whole face can become a mass of scar tissue with this process.

Because of the dangers of this type of deep peel, cosmetologists now offer a *mild peeling procedure*, using milder chemicals. These chemicals cause a limited amount of peeling and drying of the skin as well as some edema of the face. The peeling does not go deep enough to remove any scars, but the temporary edema puffs out and tightens the skin, making the scars seem considerably shallower. As soon as the edema wears off, usually after two to three weeks, the scars reappear exactly as they were before the mild peel. Mild peeling, while not as terribly damaging or dangerous as deep peeling, is far from innocuous. In people with thin skin it can cause scarring; if proper sterilization procedures are not followed, the raw peeled skin can develop serious infections; in addition, freshly peeled skin is extremely sensitive to sunlight and easily develops brown splotchy areas of discoloration. Finally, this procedure, which is a waste of money at any price, usually costs in the range of a hundred and fifty to two hundred dollars.

Scar removal is not the only area where dangerous or useless techniques and products are offered for acne care. For every useful treatment of acne there are probably three products or techniques that should be avoided.

Treatments to Be Avoided

The more commonly found ones to beware of are:

OATMEAL SOAP: Oatmeal soap has a soothing effect on the skin, but it does not remove the top layer of dead skin nor does it slow down the function of the skin's oil glands.

OZONE GAS: This gas is sprayed on the skin by a cosmetologist as part of a facial for oily or acned skin. It is supposed to refresh and revitalize the skin. Ozone has been shown to be an antiseptic, but alcohol is far superior, less dangerous, and much cheaper. Pure ozone is considered by the F.D.A. to be ten times more toxic than the chemical war gas phosgene.

GALVANIC CURRENT: A glass rod with a metal filament within it conducts a current that is applied to the face. The promotional material would have us believe that this current melts the oil in the follicles. There is nothing magic about galvanic current. It is no different from the current used to power your kitchen appliances. It is just as dangerous and has no place in the treatment of acne. Galvani happens to be the name of an Italian scientist who pioneered electricity, and galvanic current is simply an archaic way of saying electricity.

THE MINI VACUUM CLEANER FOR THE FACE: This is a machine that is supposed to pull out blackheads and clogged oil from the pores. It doesn't.

SEAWEED SERUM OR EXTRACT: There is no reason at all why seaweed in any form should be helpful against acne. Seaweed is used in the manufacture of cosmetics primarily as a thickener or as part of a gel mask. It has no effect on the skin.

VITAMIN E: This vitamin has recently been promoted as a miracle drug for many conditions, including acne. Let it be stated unequivocally that vitamin E has not been found to help acne. It cannot be absorbed through the skin, so that all topical applications of vitamin E do not penetrate to the problem area. Vitamin E has, on the other hand, been shown to produce severe allergic reactions in some cases. At least one product containing vitamin E has had to be withdrawn from the market because it caused so many allergies.

NATURAL AND ORGANIC PRODUCTS: As described earlier, in Chapter 2, organic and natural products have no special value. It may be nice to dream that a peach soap will give one a "complexion like a peach," but unless this soap also contains active anti-acne ingredients like sulfur or resorcinol, the acne condition will not get any better.

Useless aids that are sold for acne are not just a waste of money; they also keep people from using the most effective acne fighters, or from seeking medical help for severe acne.

Special Cases of Acne

After the early twenties acne should disappear. One or two minor spots every few months is not out of the ordinary, but constant skin breakout means that something is wrong. It could be due to mismanagement of normal or oily skin, a reaction to medication, or a glandular imbalance. Whatever the cause, it can and should be cured.

During adolescence constant and concentrated treatment is needed just to diminish outbreaks. In adult acne, the right treatment can stop acne problems, and keep them from returning.

. . .

Acne Caused by Mismanaged Skin

The most frequent cause of adult acne and the simplest to correct is mismanagement of the skin. If you are over twenty, have frequent outbreaks, and answer yes to four or more of these questions, you are probably causing your own skin problems.

A PROFILE OF ACNE CAUSED BY MISMANAGED SKIN

1. Is your acne mostly blackheads, whiteheads, and small pimples, without any large cysts?
2. Do you use a cream for cleansing?
3. Do you feel that you have "combination skin"?
4. Do you use moisturizers?
5. Did you have mild acne (or even none at all) as a teenager?
6. Are your periods regular?
7. Are you taking any medication, including birth control pills?
8. Are your pimples concentrated on the chin, jaw, and neck areas?
9. Are you between twenty-five and thirty-five?

Acne due to mismanaged skin usually arises from the unnecessary use of creams and moisturizers. Many women live in dread of dry skin, having been taught that dry skin is a sign of aging and the cause of wrinkles. If dry skin can be stopped, they feel, wrinkles can be avoided and the skin will always look firm and smooth. Although the skin is normal or only slightly oily, even the tiniest sign of tightness or flaky skin is viewed as ominous and greasy beauty aids are quickly slathered on. For instance, they might use oily cleansing creams, which remove some surface dirt and old makeup but which cannot dislodge most of the other accumulated refuse on the skin.

After this mistreatment the skin begins to look muddy and dull. All it needs at this point is a good, thorough cleansing with soap and water to remove the top layer of dead cells, oil, and dirt that have accumulated daily, but this is not to be. Misinterpreting dull skin for dry skin, these women apply a moisturizer to combat the imagined problem. This is more than the skin can endure. Already drowning under old oil and dead cells, the pores cannot cope with a new onslaught. They rebel with a profusion of blackheads, whiteheads, and pimples.

There is nothing basically wrong with the hormones or oil glands in such cases. It is simply the improper cleansing and excess creams clogging the pores that cause the acne.

In the treatment of acne caused by mismanaged skin, the aim is to reduce the acne and allow the skin to restore itself to what it would normally be—healthy, clear, and smooth.

CLEANSING:

Soap. You want a soap with good degreasing abilities, but with a lower sulfur content (no higher than 3 percent) than the one normally used for adolescent acne. One such soap is ACNE AID SOAP by Stiefel.

Washing grains. This gritty cleanser will rub the dead skin cells off the surface of the face and remove superficial scarring and skin discoloration after an acne outbreak.

OIL-BALANCE CONTROL:

Drying lotion. It should contain sulfur, salicylic acid, and/or resorcinol, just like the lotion for adolescent acne. For the first two to three weeks of use it should be worn both day and night. When the skin improves, it should be applied only at night.

TONING:

Astringent. The same type used for oily skin will do an excellent job. Remember, this type of adult acne is not as oil-troubled as adolescent acne. A too enthusiastic drying of the skin will make it rough, sore, and flaky; this is exactly the kind of skin women try to avoid by using creams to excess and thereby causing acne in the first place.

Masks. Clay-based masks are good for this type of acne. They soak up oil and, when removed, carry with them some of the caked dead skin that has built up on the face. The masks used for oily skin are an excellent choice.

Saunas. The moist heat of the saunas will melt the sebum stuck in the pores, and generally clean the face.

Cosmetics. Only oil-free cosmetics should be used at this time.

No creams and lotions of any type should be used on the face during the period of treatment for adult acne. If you have enough oil to cause pimples, you have enough oil to maintain good moisture balance on your skin.

During treatment, the skin should feel somewhat flaky and dry for several weeks until the acne is brought under control. This means you are finally ridding yourself of the layer of dead skin and grease that has been clogging up your pores. The use of creams and oils to counteract this dryness will only make the skin break out again.

A PROGRAM OF CARE FOR MISMANAGED SKIN

NIGHT

1. Make a lather of hot water and soap on your hands, and spread it on the face, rubbing all the areas on the face gently but firmly. If the lather begins to dry out, work up a fresh lather in your hands and apply it once again.

2. Rinse with lukewarm water.

3. Let your face dry in the air.

4. Give yourself a hot-pack treatment as described on page 56, or use a facial sauna.

5. With a cotton ball swab the astringent on your face. Do not rub it in; just smooth it on.

6. Again let your skin dry in the air.

7. Spread a layer of acne lotion over the affected areas, not just on each pimple, but over the entire affected skin.

DAY

Follow the same procedure described for night care for two to three weeks. Then omit drying lotion during the day. It is very important that you use oil-free makeup, since this type of acne is caused in large part by the application of oil-rich products. Make sure that your foundation is really oil free, not just one that calls itself "medicated." They are not the same thing at all. "Medicated" means that it contains something like sulfur or alcohol. "Oil free" means that it has no oil to clog up your pores.

TWICE-WEEKLY DEEP-CLEANSING

Twice a week, instead of your usual nightly care, the following should be done to treat your acne thoroughly (more frequent use of this program may lead to irritation of the skin).

1. Wash with acne soap.

2. Wash with scrubbing grains.

3. Apply hot towels for five minutes.

4. Rinse your face in cool (not cold) water. Cold water will be too much of a shock for the skin and may break some blood vessels.

5. Apply a clay mask and leave it on for thirty minutes.

6. Wash off the mask with cool water; dry your face.

7. Apply an astringent.

8. Apply a medicated acne lotion.

Dry-skin Acne

Another somewhat rare type of adult acne is found in people with dry skin. This seems like a contradiction in terms, since acne is basically caused by excess oil, and dry skin, by definition, does lack the normal amount of oil. But in dry-skin acne, even tiny amounts of oil can cause acne problems. This could be the result of the size and shape of the pore follicle itself. A long thin follicle makes it difficult for the oil to reach the surface, and the trapped oil forms a whitehead. Dry-skin acne can also arise if the small amount of oil produced by the oil gland is particularly rich in fatty acids.

Because this type of acne occurs in the same age group—twenty-five to thirty-five—as acne that results from mismanaged skin, it is important to accurately differentiate the two, since they require very different types of care.

. . .

A PROFILE OF DRY-SKIN ACNE

1. You had little or no acne as a teenager.

2. Your skin has been fairly dry since adolescence.

3. You have dry hair (this is a vital point, since most true cases of youthful dry skin are always accompanied by dry hair).

4. You have regular periods.

If this profile accurately describes your skin history, the best way to deal with your acne is with low dosages of a tetracycline. This antibiotic changes the chemistry of the oil produced by the follicles so that they no longer form whiteheads.

Tetracycline is available only by prescription, and if you have this kind of acne you must see a dermatologist for treatment.

Dry-skin acne cannot be treated with the usual anti-acne soaps and drying lotions. They would be too harsh and drying on this skin, and would make the complexion look red, sore, and flaky. So clean and tone the skin according to the standard program for dry skin, and let the tetracycline clean up the acne.

Drug-caused Acne

A less frequent but still important cause of adult acne is the use of certain medications. Medications that can cause skin eruptions include cortisone, an anti-inflammatory drug given for a wide spectrum of illnesses; INH, an antibiotic used in the treatment of tuberculosis; ACTH, a drug that stimulates the body's production of cortisone-like hormones; Dilantin, a drug given for the control of epilepsy; and last (but by no means least) birth control pills.

These medications are taken by millions of women for often serious medical problems. Acne, in this context, may be seen by your doctor as a relatively trivial side-effect of a very useful drug, and as such may be dismissed lightly. For anyone who has to live with the acne, however, this problem might not seem trivial. Ask your physician to initiate some anti-acne treatment; in the case of birth control pills, he may be able to alter the dosage or the type of pills you are taking so as to do away with this side-effect.

Acne as a complication of medication usually appears a few

weeks after the drug is started and disappears soon after the drug is withdrawn. This kind of acne usually can be controlled by following the plan outlined for adolescent acne.

Hormonal Acne

The final and most serious form of adult acne is that provoked by a glandular imbalance. There are two general forms of hormonal imbalance and these are treated differently.

The first and easiest to treat is the nonspecific imbalance. During adolescence, the glands are naturally off-balance. This does not harm the rest of the body, but merely causes acne and, occasionally, the growth of excess hair on the face. After adolescence, the hormones are usually stabilized and the acne disappears. But in some people, the glands continue to produce unbalanced amounts of hormones, and the acne persists.

The following questions will suggest whether or not you have this postadolescent type of hormonal acne.

A PROFILE OF POSTADOLESCENT HORMONAL ACNE

1. Are your periods very irregular? (The answer to this question must be yes.)
2. Did you have moderate to severe acne with cysts as a teenager?
3. Are your skin and hair both greasy?
4. Did one or both of your parents have severe acne?
5. Did your acne resist conventional treatments like acne soaps and lotions, slush baths, and/or tetracycline?

If the answer was yes to most of these questions, many doctors feel that the best way to treat this type of acne is by hormone therapy.

While there is considerable controversy about this form of therapy, these doctors feel that hormone therapy, properly administered under the close supervision of a physician, will probably alleviate and control this condition. Some doctors report that as many as 92 percent of their patients are helped.

Simply stated, hormone therapy attempts to correct the hormonal imbalance that persists after puberty by supplying the lacking hormone. This imbalance is not the same in everyone. To prescribe too little or too much of a hormone may make your acne worse or have no effect on it at all. Careful examination of your problem by your dermatologist or endocrinologist will determine the exact amount of the hormone suitable for you. All too many failures of hormone treatment for acne are not due to the hormones themselves but to the improper dosages for individual patients.

Women who are used to taking the pill for contraception may be surprised to find that the dosages used for acne control are quite different from those used for birth control.

It is dangerous to treat yourself with the high dosages of hormones that are usually required to treat acne. The best and safest way to begin this treatment is to find a dermatologist who uses this therapy for adult acne (not all do). A dermatologist will find the proper dosage for you, and, in addition, will give you a standard program of cleansing, with drying soaps, hot packs, peeling lotions, and a slightly restricted diet. He or she may also prescribe low doses of tetracycline, which, as you will recall, alters the composition of the oil glands.

After three to four months of treatment, the skin will usually be clear. There may be some residual scarring, but generally these scars will fade with time. If they do not, they can be removed —without the fear that the skin will break out again.

Some women complain of water retention from such hormone therapy. A low-sodium diet will help resolve this problem. Such a diet limits canned meats and fish, all prepared and convenience foods, pickles, luncheon meats, catsup, mustard, hot dogs, smoked meats or fish, celery, hard cheese, soy sauce, olives, sauerkraut, and shellfish. People on low-salt diets should concentrate on fresh meats, poultry, and fish, sweet butter, fresh vegetables and fruits, rice, potatoes, breads and cakes from bakeries rather than the packaged varieties (the latter contain preservatives that are types of salt, like disodium phosphate). Always read the label on prepared foods, since salt is used in many foods you would think contain no salt, as, for example, applesauce, frozen orange juice, and ice cream. If the label says sodium of any kind, put it back and look for something else. There are now many products available that are prepared without salt. Look for low-salt mayonnaise, peanut butter, mustard, catsup, cookies, cereal, tuna, and salad dressing. Never use salt in cooking or add extra salt to your food. There is enough natural salt in most foods to take care of the body's need for it.

When eating out, avoid dishes where salt is bound to be added. Pass up soups, stews, sauces, and salad dressings.

To see what a low-salt diet looks like, here is a sample menu (containing seventeen hundred calories). You can vary the calorie count by changing the portions of meat, fruit, and rice.

BREAKFAST

½ grapefruit
2 eggs, 2 slices toast, salt-free margarine, jelly
coffee or tea

LUNCH (at a restaurant)

hamburger
French fries
sliced tomato
(Remember, no catsup or mustard)

DINNER

fresh fruit cup
broiled chicken, rice, salad, green vegetable
salt-free cookies, coffee

For more diets and salt-free recipes, two very good books are: *Cooking Without a Grain of Salt* by Elma W. Bagg (Doubleday and Co., and Bantam Books) and *Everything You Want to Know About Salt-free Recipes* by Nancy Lloyd (Pyramid Publications).

Usually after about one year of successful hormone treatment, your dermatologist will begin decreasing your dosage of hormones. If all goes well, within a year or two you can be taken off medication altogether. Sometimes the skin flares up again; should this happen your dermatologist can start you on a second course of therapy. More often than not, your skin will remain clear. It may, however, be fairly oily and, if so, it must always be treated with relatively strong soaps and astringents to look its best (for details see the section "The Care of Oily Skin," pages 46–50).

The second type of adult acne resulting from hormonal imbalance is somewhat more complex. Here there is an underlying medical reason, such as ovarian cysts, an underactive thyroid, or tumors of the adrenal glands or ovaries, which causes the glands to misfunction. There is no simple profile to determine these conditions, but some of the following symptoms may point to such a problem:

1. Irregular periods.
2. Excess body hair and facial hair.
3. Obesity.
4. Severe acne that continued from adolescence to adulthood without interruption.
5. Small whiteheads, especially on the forehead and chin.
6. Difficulty in becoming pregnant.
7. Acne that resists simple treatment.

If you recognize yourself in this profile of adult acne, you should probably see an internist rather than a dermatologist. This type of acne may be the signal of a medical problem. The doctor who sees you will suggest a series of blood and urine tests to pinpoint exactly what is wrong and will indicate the necessary treatment—both for the basic problem and the existing acne.

Fortunately most forms of adult acne can be more easily controlled than adolescent acne. Once under control it frequently disappears entirely. The skin is then handled like normal or oily skin and looks clear.

5 / Problems of the Mature Skin

Fine Lines

Almost everyone over twenty-five has some lines on her face. They appear most frequently around the eyes, on the forehead, and in the cheek areas around the nose and mouth. These superficial lines can make the face seem older, tired, and drawn. However, they are not necessarily a sign of true aging, but rather they are usually an indication of wear and tear on the skin and excessive exposure to sun.

What Causes Fine Lines

The collagen fibers in the dermis (the skin's lower layer) are responsible for skin tone. Many people see the skin as something stretchy, like rubber or elastic, but in reality it is not that way at all. Visualize the skin instead as a piece of cloth like cotton or silk. Pull it one way, then the other. Notice how it changes its shape. The cloth does not grow larger, just *changes* in shape. Collagen moves and changes in the same way. The flexibility is due to the unique arrangement of its fibers: they are linked in such a way that they can bend and twist when you move your face while eating, yawning, talking, or just making a face.

All these movements pull the skin of your face into a new shape, and although the skin has quite a tolerance for returning to its usual state, after twenty-five years of almost constant motion, it begins to get weary. The collagen fibers begin to lose their wonderful ordered quality. They become frayed at the edges, and change into a more solid and less flexible mass. Returning to the cloth analogy, think of how a well-worn suit or pair of pants seems to maintain the shape of its owner even when it rests on a hanger.

In skin, the stretching and sagging first appears as fine lines around the areas where the face moves the most: the eyes, the mouth, and the forehead.

What Can Be Done About Fine Lines

The popular approach to the care of lines has been confined to slathering the skin with oil and water.

Lined skin is often but not always dry skin, skin that has lost a great deal of its natural water. This desiccated skin makes lines look much deeper. Think of a balloon. When it is empty, it looks wrinkled and lined. If you blow it up or pour water into it, the surface swells and becomes smooth and unlined. The same thing happens to skin. If you feed dry, lined skin with water-rich creams and masks, the water content will rise, and the skin will puff up, making the lines less noticeable.

Creams and moisturizers can make lines *seem* less deep but cannot prevent or permanently eliminate fine lines. These creams and moisturizers do not act on the real causes of fine lines; namely, wear and tear and sun damage.

A realistic and successful program for the prevention and care of fine lines involves three basic approaches:

1. Decreasing wear and tear of the skin;
2. Protecting collagen against sun damage;
3. Cleansing, oil-balance control, and toning, to make the lines *seem* less apparent.

DECREASING WEAR AND TEAR: The daily motions of the face can put considerable strain on the collagen fibers. Of course, you can't maintain a poker face all day long. But the awareness of what pushing your face around in all sorts of expressions can do should make you rethink some mannerisms such as wrinkling your brow, pouting, or grimacing.

Another practical way to reduce abuse of the embattled collagen fibers is to sleep face up. Look at someone while he or she is asleep. See how distorted the face looks pressed on the pillow. The pressure on the face can affect the flexibility of the skin. Try sleeping on your back for a month. You'll be amazed how much better your skin looks.

Facial exercises are actually just another form of making faces, yet women are still being solemnly advised to puff their cheeks out as full as possible; to purse their lips forward and blow the air out slowly; to roll their eyes swiftly in all directions; and to invent new ways of making funny faces. Try these "facial exercises" just once, watching yourself in the mirror as you do. See what a strain they put on all areas of your face.

The rationale behind these exercises is that they tighten up facial muscles so that the skin will be tauter. But skin tone has very little to do with muscle tone and these unnecessary facial motions increase the strain on the collagen fibers and can actually promote lines.

PROTECTION FROM THE SUN: The sun is your skin's worst enemy. The ultraviolet (uv) rays of the sun have the ability to specifically destroy collagen fibers. They change them from a loosely linked, flexible tissue to a solid mass of fragmented fiber shreds. When the collagen reaches this point, it has lost all of its ability to move properly, and lines will form. Sun damage is rapid and cumulative. The collagen fibers are so sensitive to uv rays that even on a gray winter day they can be damaged by exposure to the few rays that are available.

If you are one of those people who looks best suntanned, turn to the section on sun and the skin (pages 128–34) for a full discussion of how to minimize damage and maximize tan.

While the skin is being protected from further sun and stress damage, certain creams, masks, and other cosmetics can make the skin *appear* to be less lined and drawn.

Most of these beauty aids revolve around one of two principles. They either plump up the skin with water or they coat the surface of the skin with a flat transparent film. This smooth flat surface reflects the light more evenly than does the surface of irregular, lined skin, so that it looks as if it is less lined than it really is.

When you use these cosmetics, you are not curing wrinkles but, rather, masking their contours from view. All this is to the good, but in using such aids first be sure that you know what you are really doing to and for your face.

CLEANSING:

Cleansing creams. Lined skin is usually dry skin, and should therefore be treated in much the same way. Cleansing creams and lotions that rinse off with water are the best; they remove the dirt and debris on the skin but do not dehydrate it or remove too much oil.

Scrubbing grains in cream base. Scrubbing grains are usually reserved for oily and acned skin, where they do an excellent job of removing the top layer of cells. In their usual form they are far too drying for lined skin. However, when mixed with a washable cleansing cream, they will remove dead dull skin to make the complexion brighter and softer with no drying effects.

OIL-BALANCE CONTROL: While all creams help the skin hold water to some degree, there are some that are better than others. The better ones contain substances that hold water in the skin, either the natural moisturizing factors (N.M.F.'s) or estrogens. Estrogen creams are like N.M.F. creams in that estrogens, when applied to the surface of the skin, have the ability to attract and hold water in the skin's cells. Think of how often you retain water during your menstrual period. This estrogen-caused phenomenon that takes place throughout your body is mimicked locally when creams containing this hormone are applied to the skin. The more water the skin retains, the more the skin puffs out, making its fine lines less visible. Two products containing N.M.F.'s are SECOND DEBUT and Love's N.M.F. CREAM. Both Helena Rubinstein and Elizabeth Arden have put out an estrogen cream. This type of product is frequently called a moisturizer or moisturizing cream.

TONING:

Astringents. These can make the face seem firmer, and the pores look smaller. These effects are just illusions, since astringents create only a slight puffiness or fullness of the skin. But this action does make the skin *look* better. Choose an astringent according to the guidelines established for dry-skin astringents (page 40). Remember, when you examine a list of any product's ingredients, you are looking mainly for key chemicals. Most commercial products have a wide variety of ingredients. Look for those that give the greatest effectiveness, and avoid ingredients that can make your skin problems worse.

Masks. These are another aid. Because a mask forms a solid, watertight film on the face, while it remains there the skin accumulates a large supply of water. In addition, as a mask dries, its tightening action stimulates the circulation in the face, promoting a nice, rosy glow. When the mask is removed, it usually pulls off the top layer of the dry dead cells, giving the skin a smooth, translucent look. The end effect will be a smoother, clearer, and more attractive complexion. The best masks for lined skin are the gel types. They form a clear film that is either rinsed off with water or pulled off in one piece. These masks are made with various bases, ranging from gelatin, Irish moss, and seaweed extracts to plastic substances. Two such products are Shiseido's EXTRA RICH FACIAL PACK and BRUSH-ON PEEL-OFF MASK by Helena Rubinstein. Honey masks and those using egg whites form the same kind of films as the gel masks and are also good. Their value is based on the film-forming properties of the honey and the egg whites, and not on any special healing powers of the two natural substances themselves. Clay masks absorb too much oil from the skin to be good for lined skin.

Saunas. These are also good for lined skin. They clean out the skin, while at the same time they deliver enough water to keep it moist and soft.

Clear films. These, a wonderful new cosmetic aid for lined skin, are spread on the face under or over the makeup. The film does not change anything in the skin, but forms an invisible smooth surface on the surface of the skin that reflects light evenly and gives the face a less lined appearance. One such product currently on the market is BYE-LINES (Elizabeth Arden), which sells for five dollars an ounce.

Several years ago, many companies came out with a similar coating for the face based on bovine serum albumin—a protein extracted from cows' blood. Unfortunately, the advertising and promotional claims for these products were excessive and exaggerated, making it sound as if these products changed the skin and actually made lines less deep. The F.D.A. felt that the claims made such products sound like drugs, which have to be approved by the F.D.A. before being marketed. The F.D.A. charged that if such products were not drugs, then their advertising contained false and misleading claims, and the agency had these products removed from commercial distribution. Actually, these products were safe and effective in temporarily making facial lines less obvious. Perhaps now, with a new demand from the buying public, the manufacturers will again market such products with more judicious advertising.

A PROGRAM OF CARE FOR FINE LINES

NIGHT

1. Cleanse with a washable cream.

2. Rinse off well with lukewarm water.

3. Pat dry, very gently.

4. Apply estrogen cream or other N.M.F. moisturizer. Smooth cream all over the face. Try not to rub it in but let it sink in by itself.

DAY

1. Cleanse as at night with a washable cream.

2. Rinse off well with cool water.

3. With a clean cotton ball, apply astringent over face with a patting motion. Do not rub the ball over the face, just pat it on.

4. Let face dry.

5. Spread on a clear film if it goes on *under* makeup.

6. Apply greaseless N.M.F. or estrogen moisturizer.

7. Apply makeup foundation, eye makeup, and cheek blusher or rouge.

(8. Spread on a clear film if it goes on *over* makeup.)

WEEKLY FACIAL

1. Cleanse with a washable cleanser.

2. Steam face for five minutes.

3. Rinse with cool water.

4. Cleanse with scrubbing grains in washable cream—made by mixing one half teaspoon of a product like PERNOX or BRASIVOL with two teaspoons washable cleansing cream.

5. Rinse again with cool water.

6. Apply a gel mask; let it remain on the face for twenty minutes.

7. Rinse off the mask.

8. Apply a good moisturizer.

Things Not to Do for Fine Lines

The problem of facial lines has triggered explosions of worthless, expensive, and at times harmful beauty products and techniques. It is therefore as important to know what to *avoid* as well as what to do about wrinkles.

MASSAGE: Massage is a time-honored treatment for lined skin. It is supposed to stimulate circulation, tighten muscles, and pull the face back into line.

Actually, many dermatologists and plastic surgeons feel that massage makes lined skin worse. The pushing-pulling motion over the face creates a strain on collagen, creating a "wear and tear" situation. Instead of making the face less lined, massage can actually promote the formation of new lines.

The rubbing of cream on the face during cleansing or conditioning can cause massage-like strain on the collagen. It is another good reason to use a mild balanced soap or washable cream to cleanse the face instead of a cleansing cream.

ELECTRICAL STIMULATION: There are a number of gadgets available now in the beauty salons, or for home use, that supposedly can make the face less lined by employing electrical stimulation to make the facial muscles contract.

Unfortunately, the face is not lined because the muscles are weak and sagging, but because the collagen is out of shape. Tightening the muscles will therefore not do a thing for the collagen. In other words, these machines simply do not help.

SILICONE INJECTIONS: This is the injection of liquid silicone into some of the crevices of a line to fill it up to the level of the rest of the skin. Here is a description of the process, described by one of the most prominent plastic surgeons in the country. "I inject it very, very slowly into the skin. After each drop I rub the treated area gently but firmly to disperse the silicone droplets throughout the tissue. We don't want a solid lump of silicone embedded in the tissue. This not only looks strange, but large amounts of silicone just don't stay in one place. By dispersing the silicone droplets, we create minute tears in the tissue; the body forms internal scar tissue around each silicone droplet. This whole process creates an increased volume of tissue under the skin, and thus fills in certain types of lines."

Silicone treatments enjoyed a great popularity for several years, until some people began noticing that their improperly injected silicone traveled from its original site to other parts of the face, causing strange-looking bumps, some of which became inflamed and had to be removed surgically. Today only seven plastic surgeons in the United States are licensed to use medical-grade silicone on their patients and solely on an experimental basis (but other surgeons purify silicone for use). However, quite a few doctors feel that, properly understood and properly used, silicone might someday be a valuable cosmetic aid.

In any case, most plastic surgeons do not like to use silicone injections for fine lines because this hampers future treatment of the face. People who care enough about their appearance to have silicone injections for early fine lines will almost certainly want face lifts when their skin gets wrinkled, and face lifting will not work as well for skin that has been treated with silicone as it will for normal skin.

Sometimes, after a complete face lift, the cosmetic surgeon will touch up a few spots with silicone to perfect the appearance of the face.

ELECTRIC NEEDLES: The electric needle is used by cosmeticians and beauticians. This instrument passes an electric current through the skin and claims to cook the protein of the skin, coagulating it like an egg, and thus plumping up the skin and smoothing out the lines.

What the electric needle really does is create an irritation in the skin that causes edema, or swelling, the skin's normal response to injury, similar to the puffiness of a sprained ankle. This does plump up the skin but it means that the body has sustained a considerable assault and is reacting to protect itself. The edema goes away in a week or ten days and the skin goes back to being as lined as it was before. Although there seems to be no seriously harmful effects from the electric needle, it is very expensive; the effects that make the lines disappear are short-lived; and the constant stretching of the skin by edema can only increase the degree of skin wrinkling.

Some beauticians offer a long series of treatments with an electric needle for line removal. What happens here is that repeated electrical assaults to the skin result in the formation of fibrous tissue, or a type of scar tissue under the skin. This new growth of tissue pushes against the surface of the skin, puffing it out and taking up the slack of the skin causing the lines. After several months, the body reabsorbs this scar tissue, and the lines reappear once more.

ANIMAL-SERUM INJECTIONS: In a related treatment, animal embryo serum is injected into lines and wrinkles. This animal embryo serum is foreign protein, and as such stimulates the body to produce antibodies against it. One of the byproducts of the body's attempt to protect itself against the foreign protein is the swelling, or edema, of the irritated area. The swelling again pushes up against the skin, making the wrinkles seem to disappear. As soon as the body is satisfied that the foreign protein is destroyed, the swelling subsides, and the wrinkles reappear.

Unlike the electric needle, protein injections can have very serious side-effects. The injection of a foreign protein into your body can cause extremely virulent reactions, including hives, difficulty in breathing, or even death. This type of injection is to be completely avoided.

CHEMICAL FACE PEELING: This technique involves spreading a caustic burning solution on the face to burn away the lined skin; it has also been used for burning away acne scars and freckles. It is considered by many dermatologists and plastic surgeons to be one of the most dangerous and least successful of the cosmetic treatments currently available.

There are two basic kinds of chemical face peelings: mild superficial peeling and deep peeling, done both by beauticians and doctors.

Mild superficial peeling burns away the top layer of dry dead skin with a 10 percent solution of resorcinol, a strong caustic chemical that can dissolve skin at even a solution strength of 1 percent. The resorcinol is applied to the face with a cotton swab; there is a burning sensation, the skin turns white, then red. Within a few days a crust forms on the face; within a week to ten days this crust comes off, leaving the skin pink and firm, with the wrinkles, lines, or acne scars seemingly eliminated. But this rosy complexion is only the result of the temporary swelling of the face, a reaction to the burning effects of the resorcinol solution. When the swelling subsides in a few days or weeks, the skin looks as wrinkled or scarred as it did before the peeling.

Deep peeling burns away all of the epidermis and the very top layer of the dermis. It has been claimed that this technique not only destroys old lined skin, but, in addition, stimulates the growth of new young skin. This technique uses a combination of phenol (a derivative of carbolic acid) and croton oil, a very powerful cancer-producing drug. It is widely used in cancer research laboratories and produces malignant tumors in experimental animals after only three to four applications on an animal's skin.

One to four applications of the phenol–croton oil mixture are applied to the face. People who have undergone this treatment say that it feels like liquid fire. Sometimes the face is dusted with talcum powder to help it form a crust. At other times it is wrapped in adhesive tape to increase the burning power of the solution. The face swells considerably over the next few hours. A thick, hard crust forms on the face. One is usually confined to bed for at least a few days after such a treatment. During this time, nourishment can only be sipped through a straw, since the hard crust prevents the mouth from opening for eating.

In about ten days, the crust is peeled away, the skin underneath is a very deep red; it is sensitive, sore, and quite swollen. The lines and wrinkles are gone, but only temporarily. When the swelling subsides (usually in three to six months), the wrinkles and scars appear again.

The cosmeticians and even some doctors who do deep peeling claim that their treatments destroy wrinkled skin and generate the regrowth of young, healthy new skin. This is a dangerous half-truth. Peeling of the skin simply does *not* stimulate regrowth of firm youthful skin. The peeling is designed to be superficial (even in deep peeling). At the most it can safely take off only the epidermis and the very top layer of the dermis. Peeling of the very top layers will result in the regrowth of the same kind of tissue the skin had before. The only definite change will be the absence of freckles, brown spots, or superficial scars such as acne scars. Peeling does not affect the collagen, whose condition controls facial lines. If the peeling solutions penetrate the collagen, the skin will form an ugly scar tissue.

Even if the treatment is done by a skilled doctor, it is very difficult to control just how deep in the skin the solution will penetrate. Everyone has a different skin thickness, and even on one face some areas are thinner than others. Thus a solution that will peel off just the top layer in person A can cause scars in person B. By the same token, a solution used on different parts of person A can result in different degrees of burning.

Scarring is not the only complication you can develop from face peeling. Hyperpigmentation (splotches of dark or light coloring on the skin) frequently develops after such treatments. There have been several deaths reported after treatments with phenol solution, as a result of damage to the kidneys by phenol.

Both mild and deep peeling are expensive, painful, risky, and wholly inadequate for the removal of lines and wrinkles.

DERMABRASION: This technique of planing away the surface of the skin to remove acne scars and freckles has also been used for lined and wrinkled skin. Dermabrasion acts on the same principle as chemical face peeling (i.e., removal of the top layers of skin). Instead of using a caustic solution, dermabrasion entails the use of rapidly rotating abrasive brushes that rub off the top layers of skin. It is a much safer procedure, with much less danger of scarring and discoloration, than chemical face peeling, because it is easier to control the amount of peeling done by the brush than it is to control the amount of skin peeled away by chemicals. A skilled physician can go lightly over the areas of the face where the skin is thin and go deeper in the thicker areas. He can also use a range of fine to coarse brushes for different people and for different types of faces. This kind of variation is not possible with chemicals used in face peeling.

While it is safer than chemical face peeling, dermabrasion is just as unsuccessful in permanently removing lines and wrinkles. These problems arise deep in the collagen of the dermis, far below the level of the skin removed by dermabrasion.

Wrinkles

After the age of forty, the factors that produce early fine lines in certain areas of the face begin to accelerate their effects and start to cause deep lines, wrinkles, and sagging skin over most of the face.

The breakdown of the collagen is still a major factor in the decline of facial appearance. The aging process consists of the "hardening" of collagen so that *it can no longer resist* the daily stresses of facial motions. Sun damage continues to splinter the collagen fibers, adding to the loss of flexibility. In addition, a new problem appears: the loss of *fat pads* on the face, the distribution of fat under the skin.

The fat pads on the face have been constantly changing since infancy. Think of how round and plump an infant's face is. As you grow older you lose this "baby fat" and the face takes on more mature facial planes. Very young skin has a great deal of resiliency, so that it adjusts easily to any change in the fatty tissue distribution and the skin continues to be firm and taut over the face.

However, the underlying fatty tissue of the face starts shrinking more rapidly after age forty, actually decreasing the width of the cheeks, the chin, and the jaw area. The skin, no longer having the resiliency of youth, cannot shrink down to the now smaller face. In other words, there is just too much facial skin. The excess skin hangs in folds, giving the face a droopy look.

According to Dr. Blair Rogers, a plastic surgeon at New York University School of Medicine, some people and lifestyles are much more susceptible to wrinkles than others.

Some Factors Responsible for Wrinkles

ETHNIC BACKGROUND: People of Scottish, Irish, and English descent usually have extremely thin skin, which ages rapidly. As a rule redheaded and/or freckled individuals also have very thin skin.

DRINKING: Heavy drinking seems to age a face, particularly around the eyes. A full discussion of the effects of alcohol on the skin is found on page 136.

FACIAL EXPRESSIONS: Actors and actresses who are constantly called upon to use exaggerated facial expressions often show signs of facial aging at a much earlier age than would normally be expected. More generally, people who tend to express their feelings with changing facial expressions soon show the effects in the form of premature wrinkling.

EXCESSIVE CREAMING AND MASSAGING OF THE FACE: The constant rubbing motion of creaming is enough to cause already weakened facial collagen fibers to break and crumble. Consider the possible creams that can be used: cleansing creams to remove makeup, followed by night creams and day creams, vanishing creams, eye creams, and throat creams—all applied with a rubbing action. All this rubbing only makes the skin more wrinkled. Professional facial massage will do exactly the same thing.

FREQUENT WEIGHT GAIN AND WEIGHT LOSS: The rapid gain of ten or more pounds, followed by a crash diet to take off this weight, can cause premature wrinkling of the skin. The increase in weight pulls on the skin, stretching it to cover the newly formed fat under the skin. Rapid weight loss does not permit the tissues of even young skin to adjust to the new smaller shape of the underlying facial structures. Try to avoid weight gains, but if you do gain weight, lose it slowly at the rate of a pound or two a week at the most.

TOO MUCH SUN: Extremely wrinkled and deeply lined skin is usually the result of too much exposure to the sun. The damage done to the skin by the sun is far worse than anything natural aging or massaging can do.

SMOKING: Recently it has been shown that heavy smokers have more wrinkles than nonsmokers. The reason seems to be that smoking impairs the circulation of blood to the skin. The decreased circulation means that less food and oxygen are reaching the skin and more water and carbon dioxide are building up within the cells. This unhealthy environment for the skin contributes to wrinkling (see the photograph on page 135).

· · ·

What Can Be Done About Wrinkles

When the face has reached this degree of wrinkling and bagging, no creams, potions, extracts—or prayers—can help it. The products and programs that were used successfully against dry and lined skin cannot significantly help at this time.

Many of the useless methods promoted for lined skin (electrical stimulation, silicone therapy, face peeling, placenta extracts, just to name a few) are pushed even more strongly for wrinkled skin, but at this point, the only procedure that will improve facial appearance is cosmetic surgery.

There has been a great deal of discussion on the morality of cosmetic surgery. Opponents say it is vain and selfish of people to tie up hospital beds for beauty problems. They claim that people who want this type of surgery have childish personalities, are unable to accept old age gracefully, and are even, at times, psychotic.

Recently, however, a prominent British plastic surgeon published the results of a ten-year study of 106 patients who had undergone surgery for sagging skin of the face, eyelids, and neck. He found them to be an unusually stable group of people. Most were married, with less than 20 percent having been divorced. They were for the most part well educated, outgoing, highly active in community affairs, and many had challenging jobs. *Every* patient was very pleased with the results of the operation. They claimed to feel for the most part emotionally and physically better, and sociological study after the operation showed a remarkable spurt of emotional and social growth among these people. Over half of the group reported new jobs, a promotion or a raise, new friendships and greater emotional stability.

Simone de Beauvoir writes in the *Force of Circumstances* of the horror she feels when she looks at her face in the mirror. She cannot believe it is her own. She has a dream that she is thirty and, within that dream, she has another dream that she is fifty. When she first awakes, her immediate thought is what a horrible dream. However, she soon realizes that the dream is true, that she is old, that she is indeed fifty.

There is no need for this psychological torture. Cosmetic surgery is usually safe, effective, less expensive than a mink coat, a Volkswagen, or a two-week trip to the Caribbean, and to many people it is a new lease on life.

The basic cosmetic operation for aging is the complete face lift. This consists of lifting and smoothing the skin around the cheeks and forehead, removal of the baggy tissues around the eyes, and elimination of the loose flabby skin of the neck.

Recently some plastic surgeons have offered individual operations for specific areas of the face, such as baggy tissue around the eyes or a flabby neck. Yet many doctors feel that spot operations for wrinkles do not yield the best results in most cases. If the eye area has become baggy enough to need surgical treatment it is likely that the rest of the face needs lifting too. Merely fixing the eye area will not really improve the appearance of the face. In addition, subsequent cosmetic surgery to correct the other parts of the face might not be as successful as if all the steps had been done at one time. Finally, it is a lot more expensive to approach cosmetic surgery in this piecemeal way. The complete face lift plus hospitalization may cost several thousand dollars. It may seem much cheaper to have only the neck smoothed, for say a thousand dollars. However, subsequent operations to correct cheek wrinkles, baggy tissue around the eyes, or lined foreheads will bring the total cost of these additional operations to far more than what the complete face lift would have cost originally.

Aging skin is wrinkled and no longer lies smoothly on the face. The lift pulls up and tightens the excess skin. It does not change the basic contours of your face. The problems of changing bone structure and subcutaneous (under the skin) fat loss are not altered by this operation; your face will never again have the round contour of a young girl. After a successful face lift you will look mature, but you will look much better.

While the basic face lift follows certain set steps, each surgeon adds his own special technique. Here is a description of the technique used by one of the leading plastic surgeons in the United States.

FACE-LIFT OPERATION:
1. The hair is sectioned (parted) off around the face about one half inch back from the forehead. The hair behind and in front of this part is tied to keep it out of the way. The part line is going to be the incision line (see Diagram 6).
2. The face is swabbed with an antiseptic solution, and allowed to dry in the air.

Diagram 6.

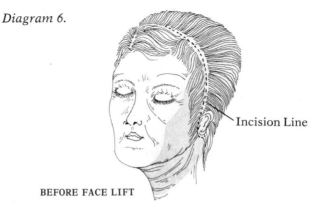

Incision Line

BEFORE FACE LIFT

3. The eye area is repaired first (see Diagram 7). A leaf-shaped section is removed from the upper lid. The edges are sewn together. The scar is in the natural fold of the eye, so it is invisible. After the top lids of both eyes are lifted, the surgeon goes on to the undereye area.

A. TIGHTENING UPPER LID

Diagram 7. Area of Excess Skin Which Surgeon Removes (The dotted lines are sewn together.)

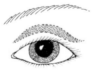

Area of Excess Skin Which Is Removed Beneath the Eye

B. REMOVING UNDEREYE BAGS

4. A second section of skin is removed from beneath the eye. The surgeon makes a tiny cut in the muscle that is revealed by removal of the skin. This is so that the surgeon can remove the excess fat pads that accumulate under the skin and make the area seem swollen and puffy. The two edges of the incision are sewn together right underneath the eye so that the scar is invisible. The eye area finished, the surgeon moves on to the rest of the face.

5. An incision is made at the scalp parting (see Diagram 8). The skin is "undermined," or lifted up from the underlying fat or muscle. This is done all around the face, going back three to four inches from the side of the face.

6. When the skin is lifted well away from the face, it is pulled up and draped over the face. The excess skin is snipped off and the skin is sewn at the incision line.

Diagram 8.

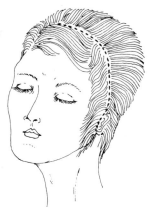

AFTER FACE LIFT

7. Cotton and gauze pads are placed over the face and eyes and the whole face (except the nostrils and mouth) is wrapped in an elastic bandage. The pads are kept in place for twenty-four to forty-eight hours, then removed.

8. After less than a week, the entire bandage is removed. The face looks a little puffy, and the eyes have bruised tissue around them. Within a few weeks, however, these signs of the cosmetic surgery disappear, and the face begins to show the improvement of the face lift.

Sometimes, after a face lift, the surgeon will also touch up a very deep line, especially around the nose or mouth, with minute amounts of silicone.

In other cases, he might perform a dermabrasion procedure to remove the top layer of mottled, sun-aged skin. In this procedure, the .skin is made firm and numb with a freezing solution. Then a vibrating wire brush is passed over the skin to remove the epidermis and the very top of the dermis. As mentioned earlier, dermabrasion is controllable, so that thin areas will be brushed more lightly than thicker ones.

Postoperative care. After a face lift certain precautions must be taken:

The face must be cleansed twice daily with a mild, neutral soap like DOVE or BASIS. Creams should not be used: The pushing and pulling motion of creaming the face puts unnecessary strain on the newly sewn tissue and can cause the skin to begin sagging once again.

One should not use dark cosmetics too soon after a face lift.

The thin scar tissue picks up and holds dye from the cosmetics, making the scar seem dark and more prominent. In addition, the dyes seem to irritate scar tissue. The scars can become very inflamed and sore. This is particularly true around the eye areas, where dark-colored cosmetics like mascara or liner are often used. This same caution should be exercised with hair dyes.

Surgeons suggest that people who ordinarily dye their hair should do so *before* a face lift so that the appearance of the hair will be good throughout the postoperative period and the patient will not be tempted to dye her hair too soon following the surgery.

Heavy false eyelashes are not to be used. They are so cumbersome and heavy that they can stretch the delicate healing eye tissue, thus making the area sag again.

Facial massage should never be applied after cosmetic surgery. It will spread the scars and make them seem broader and thicker. It will also put needless strain on newly sutured skin.

After the postoperative period, which lasts about three weeks, a woman should treat her skin in the same manner described for lined skin. With good care the results of a face lift can last for five to ten years. But, of course, during this time the aging process continues and eventually the skin will look baggy again. A face lift, however, can be successfully repeated several times during a lifetime. Although many people think that repeated face lifts will cause a mask-like expression, this is not so. Any "mask" effect is the result of overtightening the skin during the face-lift operation, meaning the operation was badly done.

As a final comment on cosmetic surgery, there is nothing noble about feeling old and ugly, and nothing evil about wanting to be beautiful and live forever.

Brown Spots, Freckles, Little Red Lines

Brown spots, freckles, and little red lines are small imperfections that can mar the mature skin and, occasionally, younger skin. They are fairly simple to deal with and their disappearance will do a lot for one's appearance.

Brown Spots

Brown spots, or liver spots, are small, flat, or slightly raised dark areas most commonly found on the face and hands. They are concentrations of melanin plus an overgrowth of skin cells. They are very shallow and lie only in the epidermis, never going deeper. They give the complexion a mottled appearance and an uneven look that seems to accentuate whatever lines or wrinkles may be on the face.

Brown spots usually appear with increasing age. Blonds and thin-skinned people are particularly liable to get them. However, exposure to the sun seems to be a determining factor in their development. Even young women in their late twenties will develop brown spots if they are sun worshippers. The appearance of brown spots in a young person indicates severe and prolonged overexposure to the sun and may indicate an increased likelihood of that person contracting skin cancer.

If someone has only a few brown spots, these can be burned off with an electric needle, similar to the electrolysis needle. An electric current passes through the needle and burns away the discolored skin. A scab forms over the treated area. When this scab falls off, the skin underneath is generally clear and smooth. This treatment should be performed only by a physician.

If there are many brown spots on the face, it is possible to remove them by dermabrasion, or with a mild superficial chemical peel, using resorcinol or salicylic acid. A brown-spot condition is one of the few that respond well to the superficial chemical peeling. Of course, this procedure should be very carefully done.

Brown spots will not return as long as the skin is protected from exposure to the sun. This means absolutely no sunbathing, and one should wear some protective shield on the face at all times. This can be a standard sun-blocking agent, such as SKOLEX by Williams, or a foundation that contains a sun-blocker, such as ULTIMA CREME MAKE UP FOR SENSITIVE SKIN by Revlon.

Freckles

Freckles are clusters of cells that have accumulated too much melanin, the dark pigment of the skin. They usually appear in childhood and persist until late middle age.

You will recall that melanin is produced in a special type of cell called a *melanocyte* (see Diagram 2, page 4). A melanocyte has a very unusual shape: it has a central body with many hollow arms extending from its sides and resembles a small octopus. Using these hollow arms, the melanocyte takes hold of an ordinary skin cell and injects a chemical substance into it that, in the presence of sunlight, becomes the brown pigment melanin. The injected cells now have the ability to produce melanin. They need only sunlight to make them go into action.

Sometimes several of the cells that have been injected with the melanin-producing substance happen to be next to one another in the skin. When the skin is exposed to sunlight these cells produce melanin and a freckle appears. Scientists do not yet know why, but the potential to develop a freckle in this area always exists. Sun will merely make the freckles visible.

Freckles can look charming scattered across the nose and cheeks, but a heavy covering of freckles can be unattractive. These freckles are best treated with dermabrasion or a mild superficial chemical peel. They will return again if the skin is exposed to the sun. Therefore, a freckled girl should be extremely careful about always wearing a sunscreen preparation, the same kind advised for brown spots. She should limit her exposure time to the sun, avoiding any serious sunbathing.

Commercial bleaching creams, lotions, and masks advertised as freckle-removers have very little value. They contain either lemon extracts or mercury compounds. Lemon has merely a small bleaching power. Mercury, although it has a much better ability to dissolve melanin, is extremely irritating to the skin. Many allergic reactions have been reported from compounds containing mercury, so it would be wise to avoid them.

Little Red Lines

Small red lines around the nose or cheek areas are the result of tiny broken blood vessels. Nobody knows exactly what causes these little red lines, or telangectasias, as they are called medically. There are, however, certain underlying factors that seem to play a large role in the disruption of these blood vessels. These include the following: heavy drinking, constant exposure to excessive warmth, high blood pressure, pregnancy, and trauma.

HEAVY DRINKING: Alcohol dilates the blood vessels of the skin. Large amounts of alcohol are thought to make them expand so much that they burst. They then will appear in the skin as small, red lines.

CONSTANT EXPOSURE TO EXCESSIVE WARMTH: Small, fragile blood vessels can rupture if exposed to a concentrated source of heat, such as an open fire or a stove. Many professional chefs have these red lines on their faces because of the long hours that they spend over hot stoves. Englishwomen also seem to be affected by these little red lines, perhaps because without central heating they must sit close to a fire or an electric heater in order to keep themselves warm.

HIGH BLOOD PRESSURE: This condition is associated with very strong pounding of the blood through blood vessels. This pressure is often high enough to burst the smaller and weaker of these vessels.

PREGNANCY: The strain of carrying the baby during pregnancy can cause poor circulation of the blood to the lower part of the body in pregnant women. This strain places additional pressure on the blood vessels of the legs. Such pressure can cause varicose veins as well as damage to the smaller blood vessels, which results in fine red lines on the legs.

TRAUMA: A heavy blow to the skin can break the small blood vessels. Breakage can also occur if constant pressure and pulling is exerted on the facial skin, as with massage.

Physicians can cauterize, or seal off, the broken blood vessels. Once these vessels are sealed, blood can no longer flow through them—it is actually the blood flowing through the damaged, dilated blood vessels that causes their red color. The physician applies an electric needle to the end of the small red line. This seals off the vessel, and the visible lines disappear. It is quite painless and relatively inexpensive.

Remember, however, that little red lines will continue to crop up at other untreated places for as long as the conditions that helped cause them in the first place still exist. Therefore, if you want to do away with little red lines permanently, then before starting cauterization treatments, you should first make sure that the underlying aggravating factors (such as heavy drinking, excessive warmth, high blood pressure, etc.) have been determined and eliminated.

6 / Cosmetic Surgery: Features to Fit Your Face

Recently there was a television program about an extremely ugly girl who was transformed into a raving beauty after cosmetic surgery. While it was a very funny and poignant program, it pointed up a common misconception about cosmetic surgery. The goal of such surgery is not to change one's face beyond recognition but, simply, to make the existing features more attractive.

There is no ideal shape and size of a nose or chin that must be attained before one has an esthetically pleasing face; it is all a matter of proportion. Unfortunately, many people go to surgeons and ask for an "Elizabeth Taylor mouth," or a "Robert Redford nose," or whatever is the fashionable feature of the day. There is no guarantee that such features would enhance those people's appearance. The desired nose might be too small, or the chin at too great an angle to be attractive on that particular face.

While there are no compulsory features, there is a series of proportions and angles for the face that have been held attractive through thousands of years of Western civilization. While the styles of fashion have changed radically, these angles and proportions have changed very little through the centuries.

Examine the pictures of these three pieces of sculpture below. The first is the head of Rameses II, who reigned as the pharaoh of Egypt some twelve hundred years before the birth of Christ; the second is a fifteenth-century statue generally attributed to Leonardo da Vinci; the third is the head of the modern American painter Georgia O'Keeffe, done by Gaston Lachaise in 1927.

Study the proportions of the forehead, the nose, and the

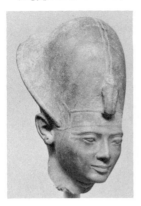

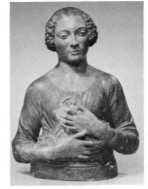

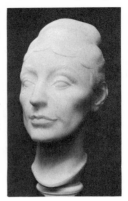

"THE LADY
WITH THE PRIMROSES"
(Italian, 1475)

mouth. They are all evenly spaced. Each section represents approximately one third of the face. The nose lines are straight, without bumps or humps. The eyes are well spaced. It is interesting to note that while the faces have similar proportions, they are quite different in appearance.

These proportions were worked out diagrammatically by a nineteenth-century sculptor as an aid for art students. These facial breakdowns have been adopted by many plastic surgeons as an aid in their evaluations of people slated for cosmetic surgery.

Diagram 9.

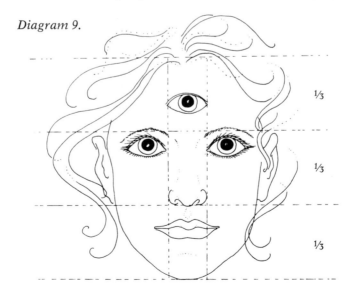

⅓

⅓

⅓

"IDEAL" PROPORTIONS OF FACE

Diagram 9 (page 100) shows the "ideal" proportions of the face. Remember, however, that these represent an average; there is considerable leeway in the proportions that make an attractive appearance. But any major deviation from these normal ranges will result in a much less appealing face.

According to these ideal proportions, the center of the nose should be directly in the center of the face. The distances from the hair line to the bridge of the nose and from the tip of the nose to the end of the chin should be equal.

At the same time, the inner corner of each eye should be in a straight line with the outer edge of the nostril. The space between the eyes should be equal to the length of one eye.

The angles at which the nose and the chin project from the face are also important to its attractiveness. Look at the diagram below.

The angle at which the nose meets the forehead (angle A) should be somewhere between 125 and 135 degrees. Smaller than 125 degrees, the nose can seem too flat. Greater than 135 degrees, it might seem to protrude too much.

The angle your nose makes with the plane of your face (angle B) should be about 25 to 35 degrees, depending on the length of the nose, the shape of the forehead, and the angle of the chin. Angles outside of this range usually produce an unattractive nose.

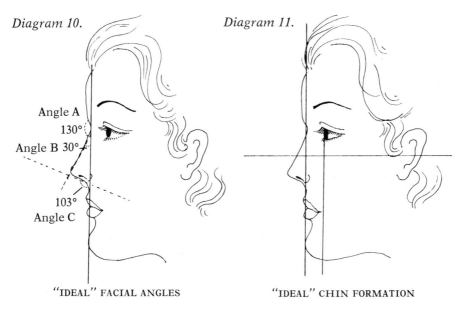

Diagram 10.

Angle A
130°
Angle B 30°

103°
Angle C

"IDEAL" FACIAL ANGLES

Diagram 11.

"IDEAL" CHIN FORMATION

Angle C, the angle at which the nose meets the upper lip, should range from 90 to 105 degrees. Less than 90 degrees can give the nose a droopy and/or long look. Angles of more than 105 degrees will make the nose appear too uplifted.

The chin must also form certain angles to be of the proper proportions for a given face. A line should run straight from the bridge of the nose to the chin. If the chin is behind this line, it is too small for the face. If it protrudes beyond this line, the chin is too large for the face.

A surgeon will frequently incorporate these diagrammatic proportions into his analysis of a facial *cephalogram*. This is an X-ray of the facial profile that shows both the bone and the soft-tissue structures. These visual devices help him decide how to bring the features into more harmonious proportions and make a face more attractive.

The Kinds of Facial Problems That Can Be Helped

There are many kinds of beauty problems that can be helped by cosmetic surgery. This chapter concentrates on some of the more common ones to illustrate the principles of facial angles and feature proportion, and to demonstrate the kind of changes that skillful cosmetic surgery can accomplish.

Usually, there is more than one problem to be corrected. However, I have divided the major problems into categories in order to discuss the various kinds of situations, and what cosmetic surgery can do for them.

Problem 1: Humped Nose, Receding Chin

This is one of the most frequent beauty problems. Correcting only one of these features will not make much of an overall improvement in the face. However, a *rhinoplasty* to reshape the nose and a *mentoplasty* chin implant to bring the chin into line

Diagram 12.

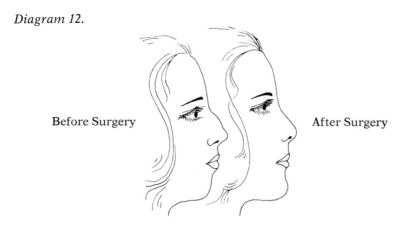

Before Surgery   After Surgery

HUMPED NOSE, RECEDING CHIN

with the rest of the face will result in a remarkable change in the appearance of the entire face.

The "Before Surgery" face (above) is a good example of this type of problem. The nose is bumpy. It protrudes from the face at an angle greater than ideal range. The chin line falls behind the meridian line, indicating that the chin is too small for the face. Cosmetic surgery smoothed out the bumps on the top of the nose, decreased the angle the nose formed with the face, and balanced these changes with a slight tilt to the end of the nose. The chin was filled out with silicone to make the jaw line stronger and to bring it into proportion with the rest of the face.

A small chin is found more frequently than a large one. If the chin is only slightly recessed, a small amount of silicone can be injected into the chin tissues to fill them out.

If the chin is moderately recessed, a silicone implant can be introduced into the chin. An incision is made inside the mouth, between the lip and the teeth (or, alternatively, the incision is made externally under the chin). The silicone implant is then sewn into the tissues. With either method, the implant brings the chin into a good line with the rest of the face.

In extremely recessed jaws the bone structure of the jaw has to be realigned. The bones are shifted and moved forward. This is a complicated operation and involves rather recent surgical techniques. It is usually performed by an oral surgeon rather than by a plastic surgeon. This kind of operation can produce an incredible change in facial appearance.

Many people have ignored chin proportions in their concern with nose shapes and sizes. Corrections of the nose are ten times as frequent an operation as corrections of the chin. This is in a sense unfortunate, since many facial problems cannot be corrected by the reshaping of the nose alone.

Problem 2: Hook Nose

The large hook nose in the picture below is another extremely frequent facial problem.

Diagram 13.

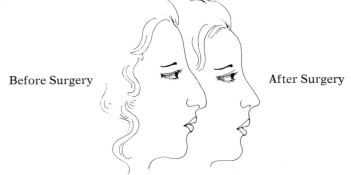

Before Surgery   After Surgery

HOOK NOSE

The excess bony tissue that makes the hump is taken out and the bridge of the nose is diminished by cosmetic surgery. In many plastic surgery situations, such noses are not shortened because it is only the angles of projection—and not the length of the individual noses—that cause the disproportion. At other times, however, this type of nose itself is too long for the face.

Problem 3: Long Nose

The problem with this type of nose is that it is too long for its face. According to the ideal reference diagram (page 100), the long nose is more than one third the total length of the face. Angle C between the tip of the nose and the upper lip is less than 90 degrees.

This problem is corrected, surgically, by removing both bone and cartilage from the nasal structure.

Diagram 14.

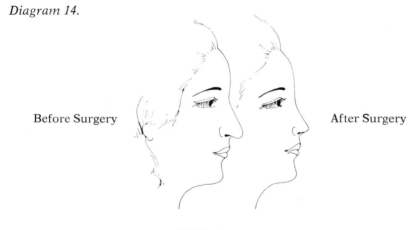

Before Surgery   After Surgery

LONG NOSE

Problem 4: Thick-tipped Nose

The width of the nose at its tip is too great in relation to its length and the arrangement of the other features of the face. This is one of the most difficult problems to correct.

The other problems of nose shape mentioned are primarily those of bony tissue. The bone can be removed cleanly and the nose will follow the line of the reduced or altered bone foundation.

A thickened tip, however, is made up mostly of cartilage, a much softer substance than bone, and it is hard to cut and shape correctly.

The appearance of every nose after cosmetic surgery depends in large degree on the personal healing patterns of an individual as well as on the way the operation was done. These factors are particularly important in the surgery performed to correct a thick tip. A poorly done operation or healing problem can result in too short a nose, or one that is strangely shaped. For this reason, it is important that this type of nose be carefully evaluated before undergoing surgery.

In thick tip situations, if the nose is not too long or too large for the face, if the bridge is fairly straight and at a good angle, and if in the final analysis the only problem is a thickened tip, it might be better to leave the nose alone. This is particularly true if the nose is short and/or the skin is thick and oily.

A short nose leaves very little margin for error. If the carti-

Diagram 15.

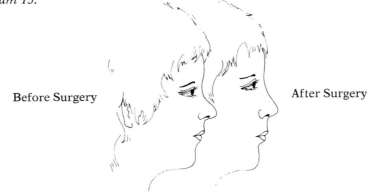

Before Surgery   After Surgery

THICK-TIPPED NOSE

lage contracts after the operation, it can result in an extremely short, thick nose. Thick, oily skin is less predictable in its recovery pattern than is thin, dry skin. It has a greater chance of rethickening during the healing process and is less likely to form a fine, delicate nose when healed after surgery.

If there are other problems present, however—if the nose is large, humped, or bumpy—then reconstruction of the whole nose will probably make a significant improvement in appearance.

Problem 5: Bumpy Nose

This nose has a bumpy, uneven surface, frequently the result of a poorly healed broken nose.

Diagram 16.

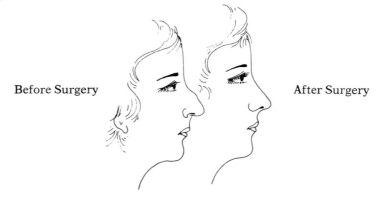

Before Surgery   After Surgery

BUMPY NOSE

The surgeon can smooth out the surface and, if necessary, remodel the tip to go with the new shape of the nose.

Problem 6: Too Large an Angle Between Forehead and Nose

This type of problem is not nearly as unattractive as a large hooked or humped nose. A tall woman with expressive eyes and a

Diagram 17.

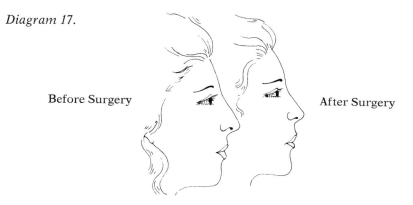

Before Surgery   After Surgery

TOO LARGE AN ANGLE BETWEEN FOREHEAD AND NOSE

good chin line could "wear" this nose with style. But in a small person, or one without other excellent facial features, such a nose might appear to be somewhat overwhelming. This type of problem frequently enjoys excellent results after cosmetic surgery.

Problem 7: Short Upper Lip

In a relaxed position, the upper and lower lip should close naturally to cover the teeth. When the upper lip is too short, the lips do not readily meet, and it is only with effort that the upper lip can descend and cover the teeth. A short upper lip is often accompanied by a nose whose shape and size could also be corrected.

Usually, the surgeon first lengthens the lip by freeing it from the *frenulum* (the membrane between the upper lip and the gum) and other soft tissues of the mouth. This allows the upper lip to meet the lower lip naturally, during relaxation.

The surgeon then corrects the shape of the nose.

Below is a before-and-after-surgery sketch of a young woman with a short upper lip and a hooked nose.

Diagram 18.

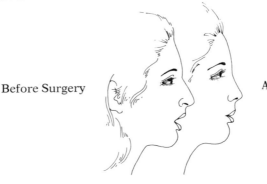

SHORT UPPER LIP, SLIGHTLY HOOKED NOSE

Problem 8: Thick Lips

Large, puffy, or protruding lips can mar an otherwise lovely face. They can be caused by allergic reactions, birthmarks, and protruding teeth, as well as by inheritance. In many cases, they can be corrected by surgical removal of excess tissue. There would be no

Diagram 19.

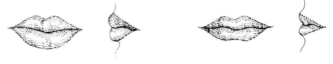

Before Surgery   After Surgery

THICK LIPS

scar, since the incision would be done inside the mouth. The diagram below illustrates the appearance of a woman with such lips before and after cosmetic surgery.

Cosmetic Surgery—
A Moral Discussion

Cosmetic surgery can bring about many changes. It can change undeniably plain facial features into definitely attractive ones. A successful change in appearance frequently leads to a positive change in personality.

Cosmetic surgery should, obviously, not be undertaken to change one's appearance for frivolous reasons. For example, if an attractive girl suddenly becomes obsessed with the shape of her perfectly acceptable nose, it might suggest that there are more psychological problems here than anatomical ones. In such cases, the desire to turn to the plastic surgeon to change one's image indicates a deep level of personal dissatisfaction that surgery could never help.

Cosmetic surgery should not be undertaken simply because "everyone else is getting a nose job." One plastic surgeon recently made the observation that an epidemic of *deviated septums* frequently hits sixteen-year-old girls of the upper middle classes. Deviated septums are internal defects of the nose that are often used as an excuse for undergoing cosmetic surgery. Plastic surgery should not be performed to change a feature to a more fashionable shape.

For every person who undergoes needless cosmetic operations, however, there are possibly a dozen people who truly need surgical help but are reluctant to obtain it. They are afraid to seem too vain, or they might be repelled by the idea of the stereotyping or standardization of an individual's face. In some instances, they are afraid they might be accused of changing their faces in order to appear more attractive sexually. They resign themselves to being unattractive and adjust their personalities and goals to their appearance. When you consider the high value our society, rightly or wrongly, places on appearance, this resignation can have sweeping effects on their emotional and professional lives.

People react positively to a pleasing face. They imbue a pretty face with a pleasant and appealing personality; a strong jaw line with a forceful personality. By the same token, people seem to take a negative, sometimes hostile, attitude toward an unattractive face. They associate a weak chin with a weak personality—and, in some strange way, people seem to act as others expect them to.

A plain girl will often respond to people's negative attitudes toward her appearance by becoming shy and withdrawn, but deep inside there is often an alive, congenial person who is dying to come out of her shell. After cosmetic surgery, such a girl will often experience a dramatic change in personality, becoming more outgoing and assertive.

Recently, in an attempt to help some women in prisons rehabilitate themselves for living in society again, a selected group of inmates was treated with plastic surgery. These women were all individuals with long criminal records and hostile personality patterns. Many of them had pronounced facial problems, such as a large nose, a tiny chin, or facial scars. What happened to many of these women after cosmetic surgery corrected their long-standing facial problems was most encouraging: In most instances, because of the new self-image the surgery had given them, they enrolled in job training courses in prison and upon release abandoned their formerly criminal and anti-social lifestyles.

The associations between sociopathic behavior and physical appearance have also been studied in men. Several years ago, it was discovered that a higher than normal percentage of male criminals had the XYY chromosome pattern in their cells (instead of the normal XXY chromosome pattern for men). It was felt, for a while, that this genetic abnormality of having an extra Y, or female, chromosome in the cells could cause the violent, often homicidal behavioral patterns observed in prisoners with the XYY chromosome condition.

However, it was also noted that the inherited XYY chromosome condition actually caused those men to grow to be extremely tall, with large, outsized noses, long chins—*and acne*. Many psychologists and sociologists pointed out that the physical characteristics of many men with XYY chromosomes caused them to experience social rejection and loneliness, and that it was this social ostracism that resulted in emotional problems, which could, as easily, have been responsible for their violent and criminal behavior.

Beauty might be skin deep—but the effects of its absence might, on the other hand, be far deeper.

7 / Skin Sensitivity

Every type of skin is potentially sensitive and may develop reddened irritated areas. This chapter deals with many of the causes of this all-too-common skin problem, as well as with methods of coping with it.

Basically the problem of skin irritation can be divided into three categories:

1. Red splotches on thin skin.
2. Skin damage by chemical burns.
3. Allergic reactions that can occur in any type skin.

Red Splotches on Thin Skin

Thin skin is an inherited trait. It is very common in red- or blond-haired people, and those of northern European descent (particularly English, Irish, or Scottish). The epidermal layer of the skin of these thin-skinned people is thinner than average, and provides less protection from surface irritation for the lower layers of the skin. At the same time, its thinness makes any changes in the skin's blood circulation much more apparent. For example, very spicy foods raise the body's temperature and slightly increase the blood circulation. In average skin, the increase in blood flow would not change the complexion. In thin-skinned individuals this change in circulation will be visible and the skin will become flushed and splotchy. The color is not evenly red because the circulation is not increased evenly. Some areas of the skin are more susceptible than others to changes in circulation.

The trick in controlling this kind of splotchiness is to avoid anything that causes increased circulation. This would include strenuous exercise, extremes in temperature (no saunas, hot packs, or icy-cold compresses), highly spiced foods (e.g., Szechuan Chinese or Mexican food), long sun exposure, yeast masks, cosmetics with mint extracts or camphor, and moderate to heavy drinking. Even two glasses of wine can cause a thin-skinned person to become flushed and splotchy.

Sometimes it is not possible to avoid these situations, and splotches appear.

First-aid Treatments

When splotches appear in thin-skinned women, there is one treatment for dry/normal skin and another for oily skin.

A TREATMENT FOR DRY/NORMAL SKIN

1. Cleanse gently your face with solidified mineral oil like ALBOLENE CREAM or baby oil.

2. Rinse well with tepid water. Let dry.

3. Smooth on a soothing cream, which contains anti-inflammatory substances like zinc oxide, cod-liver oil, allantoin, or vitamins A and D. A good example is A AND D OINTMENT by White.

A TREATMENT FOR OILY SKIN

1. Wash with a mild soapless cleanser such as DOVE by Lever Brothers or LOWILLA by Westwood.

2. Rinse well with tepid water. Let dry.

3. Make up a Burrow's solution. This is a mixture available from the drugstore—it is made by Dome Pharmaceuticals and packaged under the name of DOMEBORO POWDER. It contains boric acid, aluminum sulfate, and calcium acetate. The powder comes in little packets; dilute according to instructions.

Soak a cotton pad in this freshly prepared solution, and

apply to all the affected areas of the skin for fifteen minutes. Every five minutes resoak the cotton to freshen the solution on the pads.

4. Rinse your face with tepid water.

5. Let dry. Do not put on any harsh astringents or drying lotions for at least six hours. Use makeup lightly but do not rub the skin of your face.

Skin Damage by Chemical Burns

Certain substances will injure the skin of any person who comes in contact with them. This reaction is not an allergic one and is due simply to the irritating nature of the substance in question. These injuries are called chemical burns and are like those caused by a true burn.

Strong acids and alkalies, high concentrations of phenols and resorcinol, and mercury compounds produce this kind of reaction on normal healthy skin.

The skin must be treated with anti-burn measures in much the same way that true heat burns are managed.

Allergic Reactions

The next cause of splotchy skin is a true allergic reaction.

Many people who have allergic skin reactions have other allergies, such as hay fever, allergic asthma, "stuffed nose syndrome," or eczema. Their reactions to specific substances are allergic responses, as opposed to a reddening of the skin from a caustic irritant or an increase in blood circulation in a thin-skinned person.

Just what is happening to the body when the skin erupts with pink spots or scaly itchy areas?

An allergy is an overreaction of the body to a substance. It is a protective reaction against something it feels is threatening the body, although the substance causing the allergy may not really be toxic. With few exceptions, those substances causing allergies are not found naturally in the body, and the body simply understands that a foreign agent is present, against which it must rally its defenses to protect itself from harm.

No one becomes allergic to something the very first time he or she comes in contact with it. It takes a while for the body to build up defenses against the real or imagined danger. An allergic reaction could develop the second time one is exposed to the substance, or it could take years of repeated exposure for enough sensitivity to the substance to build up to produce an allergic reaction.

The length of time it takes to develop sensitivity depends on the kind of chemical, how much is given at each time, and how the substance enters the body. Something injected, such as penicillin, will cause a much earlier sensitization (development of allergy) than something rubbed on the skin, like a hand cream. The time of sensitization also depends on how allergy-prone the person is. Some people become sensitized much more easily and quickly than others.

There are two basic kinds of allergies, acute and delayed, and both can cause beauty problems.

Acute Reactions

Acute reactions occur within seconds or minutes after the substance comes into contact with the sensitized body. The allergen (the chemical or other substance causing the allergy) can be injected, such as various drugs; inhaled, like hair sprays or plant pollens; eaten, like strawberries; or absorbed through the skin, like house paint or face creams.

The reactions will often be related to the way the allergen was introduced into the body. Injected substances in general cause the severest allergic reactions. One can in fact develop severe breathing problems and heart failure, and even die, as a result of these allergies.

Inhaled allergens often cause sinus problems, runny noses, watery eyes, and scratchy throats.

Food allergens usually cause digestive upsets and/or hives. Hives are red raised areas on the skin that can vary in size from a tiny dot to several inches in diameter. These splotches feel warm and itchy. Hives are also the most frequent manifestation of acute allergies to something in contact with the skin.

In an acute reaction the first exposure to a substance makes the body produce *antibodies*, which are body chemicals specifically designed to repel future invasions by the same foreign substance. When enough antibodies build up, they combine with the allergen. This combination signals certain cells in the body to produce *histamines* and other histamine-like substances.

Histamines are chemically active compounds that provoke either localized or widespread changes in blood circulation. When these changes in circulation are concentrated in the skin, they produce a disruption whereby blood vessels in different localized parts of the body leak out some of their fluid content. The accumulation of this fluid under the skin produces a raised, red, itchy splotch known as a hive.

Because the reaction happens so quickly after the allergen comes in contact with the body, it is fairly simple to figure out what caused the allergic reaction. The best way to prevent any reaction from recurring is to stay away from the offending substance. In cases where it is very hard to avoid the substance, a series of shots can be given to try to diminish reactions to the allergen.

These injections contain progressively greater quantities of the specific substance to which you are allergic. When your body is exposed to the allergen in this manner, it develops what physicians call blocking antibodies. These are antibodies that combine with the offending agent, but, unlike the allergy-producing antibodies, this combination does not stimulate the body to produce histamine. As long as these blocking antibodies are present, they protect you to a greater or lesser extent against the substances that would normally cause you to produce histamine, and therefore the allergic reaction.

These blocking antibodies slowly disappear after your series of shots is completed, and must therefore be restimulated by booster shots at regular intervals for the benefits to persist.

If by chance you eat certain foods or use certain creams that cause an allergic reaction, an often effective way to stop this reaction is to take antihistamine pills. These are drugs that nullify the effects of histamines, those chemicals causing the blood vessels to leak fluid out. Without histamines, the allergic reaction often diminishes rapidly. Splotches will disappear in minutes, as will other symptoms.

Antihistamines are inexpensive drugs usually available by prescription by your physician. They are relatively safe, and are included in several over-the-counter drugs, as well.

While some acute allergic reactions disturb the skin, most skin allergies are of the second kind of reaction, called the delayed allergic reaction.

Delayed Reactions

Delayed allergy is a reaction that occurs hours or days after the allergen was introduced into the body. When this reaction involves the skin, through direct contact with the allergen, it is called *contact dermatitis*. Almost all the allergies to cosmetics are of this type. Fabrics, household detergents, and paints can also cause contact dermatitis. The skin eruptions can range from tiny pink, flat spots to angry, red, scaly patches covering large areas of the body.

As with acute reactions, one never reacts the first time one is exposed to the offending substance. During the first exposure, the body's white blood cells learn to recognize this agent as foreign. In succeeding exposures, the white blood cells rush to attack the "foreign invaders." During this period, the skin becomes inflamed, red, and itchy or even painfully sore.

During this struggle the blood vessels in the affected area of the skin become clogged with debris, which causes the skin to die; the result is flaking and scaling.

The Care and Control of Contact Dermatitis

Control of contact dermatitis involves two steps:
1. Immediate action to heal the inflamed skin.
2. Discovery of the allergy's cause.

Stopping the irritation usually begins with a moratorium on all cosmetics. Use only specially formulated soap like LOWILLA by Westwood or AVEENO by Cooper. These are extremely mild soaps with an acid pH. Aveeno contains oatmeal, which has a soothing action on the skin, and is specifically designed to be nonirritating.

Reducing the inflammation is done by bathing the skin with a cool, soothing solution. Many dermatologists prescribe some form of the classic Burrow's solution, like DOMEBORO POWDER. This creates a mildly acidic water-based liquid that contains boric acid, aluminum sulfate, and calcium acetate.

To use Burrow's solution, a cotton pad is dipped into the solution and then dabbed on the face. It should be applied twice a day for ten to fifteen minutes at a time, resoaking the cotton pad frequently.

Cortisone and cortisone-like medications are useful in a wide variety of allergy problems. They suppress many of the fundamental mechanisms of an allergic reaction. In acute reactions, the cortisones suppress the formation of antibodies and also act to minimize the inflammation.

In delayed reactions, cortisone will suppress the activity of those white blood cells that react to the presence of the "foreign" substance to which one is allergic.

In either reaction, cortisone can be used in both ointment and pill forms, depending on the severity of the reaction. Cortisones are obtainable only by a doctor's prescription, and should always be taken under medical supervision.

Antihistamines, so useful in acute allergic reactions, are not effective in delayed reactions, where white blood cells, *not histamines*, cause the inflammation and redness of the reaction.

If you have any allergy-based skin problems, the only way to prevent them from constantly returning is to learn what causes them. Repeated bad eruptions can lead to scarring of the skin. However, the discovery and identification of what is causing any given allergy can present somewhat of a problem. There is often such a long delay between the time an allergen comes into contact with the skin and the appearance of the eruptions that it is difficult to immediately pinpoint the offending chemical.

The first clue to the identity of a chemical allergen lies in the area where the red spots or eruptions originally appear. If they show up first on the hands, this would suggest soap, a household cleaner, or a hand cream. If they appear for the first time on the body, this would point to a bath soap, a body cream, clothing (the fabric itself or the fabric dye), bath powder, or bath salts. Eruptions on the face cast suspicion on cosmetics; around the eyes, eye makeup might be the culprit; a lipstick or lip gloss would be the prime suspect if the eruptions first showed around the mouth. If the eruptions appear originally on the ears, they could suggest that you are allergic to the metal in a particular pair of earrings, or to perfume dabbed behind the ears.

The next step in the detection of a guilty allergen is to

check out each suspect substance, usually by an allergist or derma-tologist, with a series of patch tests. In this procedure, the physician places a small amount of the possible allergen—say a household cleaner or a cosmetic—on the gauze side of a square Band-Aid, and then tapes it to a freshly washed area of the patient's back. A single patch for each individual substance is used, and what goes on each patch is carefully recorded, so that the doctor knows what product each patch represents.

All products used in that area must be examined. People often think it is the new product they have just tried that causes their skin irritation. This is not necessarily always so. Remember, you can develop an allergy to a given substance even if you have used it for years without suffering any reactions.

These test patches are left on the skin for twenty-four to forty-eight hours. Then they are removed and the skin examined. The area or areas that now show redness are spots where an allergic reaction has probably taken place. It can now be assumed that you are allergic to something in the product on that bandage. It may not be the entire product that is causing the reaction, however, but one or more of the many ingredients of which it is made. If you are allergic, for example, to the cream eye shadow on the test patch, it could be an allergy to the dye alone, or the perfume, or the cream base.

Here is a list of chemicals that dermatologists have found are most frequently implicated in reactions and eruptions of this kind:

SOME COMMON CAUSES OF CONTACT DERMATITIS AND WHERE THEY ARE FOUND

ALLERGEN	COSMETICS, HOUSEHOLD PRODUCTS, ETC.
1. Aluminum salts	Deodorants; antiperspirants; astringents
2. Aniline dyes	Hair dyes; eyebrow pencils
3. Ammoniated mercury	Freckle creams; antiseptic ointments
4. Ammonia	Bleaches; household cleansers
5. Barium salts	Depilatories
6. Betanaphthol	Freckle creams

7. Boric acid	Lipsticks; baby skin creams and lotions
8. Cresylic compounds	Household antiseptics
9. Essential oils (including almond, bay, bergamot, clove, lemon, orange, wintergreen, etc.)	Perfumes; deodorants
10. Formaldehyde	Plastics; preservatives; air-fresheners; disinfectants; nail hardeners
11. Lanolin	Face creams and lotions; hair preparations; skin softeners
12. Lauryl alcohol sulfates	Water-soluble preparations; cleansing creams; shampoos; body, hand, and skin lotions
13. Mercuric bichloride	Freckle creams, antiseptic lotions
14. Resins	Plastics; drip-dry clothing; Balsam of Peru; hair spray; nail polish
15. Phthalates	Insect repellants
16. Phenylenediamine compounds	Eye shadows; eyelash and eyebrow coloring cosmetics; hair colors
17. Para-aminobenzoic acid	Sunscreen lotions and creams
18. Phenyl salicylates	Suntan lotions and creams and sprays
19. Propylene glycol	Water-soluble creams; hand creams
20. Salicylic acid	Face-peeling compounds; dandruff shampoos; acne lotions and soaps; corn removers
21. Sulfur	Dandruff shampoos; acne preparations
22. Soaps	Cleansing creams; shampoos
23. Thioglycolate	Cream rinses; body builders for the hair; wave-set lotions; permanent hair-waving lotions; shampoos
24. Zinc salts	Astringents; deodorants

SOURCE: *Cutaneous Reactions to Cosmetics*, Comm. on Cutaneous Health & Cosmetics: AMA, 1965 (Lubowe, 1965; Fisher, 1970).

While cosmetics companies try to play down the problem of cosmetic allergies, it is obvious from the list of possible allergens that a bad reaction to a cosmetic can be a very real possibility for many people. Although many cosmetic allergies occur in allergy-prone people, special factors may increase the chances of an allergic reaction in usually non-allergic individuals.

Hormonal disturbances such as diabetes or thyroid deficiency, or bacterial or viral infections can change the body chemistry enough to make it react to cosmetics. Emotional disturbances can cause so many changes in the body chemistry that they often trigger allergic and other types of skin eruptions.

If the pH (acid–alkaline balance) of the skin is changed, and the skin's normal acid mantle is disturbed, cosmetic reactions can occur more frequently. In people with dry skin, the acid mantle is disturbed by using cleansing creams and face lotions that contain soap. After cleansing your face with these products, you are left with an alkaline film that disrupts your natural acid mantle for a long time. Washing with mild soap also disturbs the acid mantle, but soap remains on your face for a very short time and then is rinsed off, permitting the acid mantle to reform quickly. With long-lasting creams and lotions containing soap, the mantle simply does not have a chance to rebuild itself.

People who have oily skin can destroy their acid mantle by frequent washings with strong soap. Washing three or four times a day just does not give the skin time to reform its acid mantle. These strong soaps and frequent washings remove all the oil from the skin's surface. This severe defatting of the skin predisposes the skin to cosmetic allergies and irritation. To protect against such conditions your astringent should be as acid as possible.

Avoiding Cosmetic Allergies

It is fairly difficult to find a safe replacement for cosmetics to which you are allergic. For example, if it is determined by patch tests that you are allergic to the perfume in an eye shadow, then the chances are that most other kinds of eye shadow put out by the same manufacturer will have the same perfume and will cause the same reactions on your skin. The solution in this case is simple: switch to another manufacturer's line. However, if it is the dye or other chemicals in this eye shadow that cause a bad reaction, switching manufacturers will not guarantee an eye shadow that will not cause the same reaction. This is because many manufacturers consign the production of a cosmetic to the same outside factory and simply market the finished product. For example, the F.D.A. recently seized an eyebrow pencil for having coal tar dye in its formula. The eyebrow pencil was produced by a single factory in Tennessee but marketed in the different packages, and under the individual labels, of Avon, Hazel Bishop, Max Factor, Revlon, and Helena Rubinstein at prices ranging from 29 cents to $1.50. A similar situation was discovered after seizure by the F.D.A. of a brown eye shadow contaminated with bacteria; this product, made by a subcontractor named Oxzyn Co., Inc., was packaged for sale by Dorothy Gray, Givenchy, and Westmore. Many of the most commonly used cosmetics (just as with automobile tires, electrical appliances, and other consumer goods) are made by one source for many brand names. This practice does not affect the quality and the safety of these products; it does, however, make you think a bit when you realize that you can buy the identical cosmetic at prices ranging from 39 cents to $7.50.

Besides being sometimes vastly overcharged, if you are allergic to one eye shadow or lipstick packaged by Company X, you stand a chance of being equally allergic to the eye shadows and lipsticks marketed under the labels of Company Y, since the products of both companies can be identical.

This situation is further complicated by the fact that many products are remarkably similar in formulas from one company to another even when they are made by different factories. Most cosmetic formulas are fairly standard. They use much the same materials and processes to produce competitive goods. And it is these self-same materials to which you might be allergic in the first place.

Until very recently it was almost impossible to find out exactly what chemicals were put into a cosmetic product. Cosmetic manufacturers guarded their formulas closely. If a physician requested a full list of the ingredients in any single cosmetic, the company sent him a set of number-coded (but otherwise unidentified) patch tests in which each square of bandage was impregnated with one of the ingredients. These had to be applied to the patient to determine which chemical in the product caused the allergic reaction. The doctor would then report to the manufacturer the code number of the test patch that caused positive skin signs of allergy—

and the manufacturer, in turn, would identify only these allergenic chemicals. It was a matter of several weeks before a woman would know if she was allergic to, let us say, the lauryl alcohol sulfates found in many shampoos, lotions, and cleansing creams. This delayed knowledge of the cause of her allergy to one product was absolutely worthless in protecting her from allergic reactions caused by the presence of the same allergen in other products, since until recently very few cosmetic labels listed all of their ingredients. The only way a woman could learn if a product had ingredients causing her to break out in rashes and hives would be a reaction itself.

The awareness of cosmetic allergies on the part of the buying public has led to the introduction and growth of lines of hypo-allergenic and natural cosmetics and toiletries.

Hypo-allergenic Cosmetics

What does hypo-allergenic mean? The prefix *hypo* means less, so hypo-allergenic cosmetics are less allergy-producing than other cosmetics. But none of the manufacturers of the lines of hypo-allergenic cosmetics can agree on what makes a product less sensitizing.

There is a line of hypo-allergenic cosmetics put out by Revlon. These are very similar to the Moon Drops line of Revlon cosmetics; the major difference is that hypo-allergenic items are fragrance-free and they are packaged under sterile conditions.

While simply cutting out perfumes is not the whole answer, it can go a long way toward making any cosmetic less allergenic. In fact, about half of the known allergens in cosmetic products are the various fragrances used in them. The odds are high that it is the perfume causing your allergy problems.

If you like a particular cosmetic product very much, but it does create problems for you on the skin, it would make sense to find out if the same manufacturer puts out a fragrance-free version of a similar product.

Removing the fragrances, however, can still leave whole families of splotch-causing ingredients in even hypo-allergenic lines of cosmetics. To date, only two companies—Almay and Ar-Ex—substitute different raw materials for the commonly used ingredients to which many people react. These companies also give the full list of any product to physicians who request it.

INGREDIENTS NOT USED IN ALMAY PRODUCTS

Acacia
Alizarin
Alkaline earth sulfides
Alum
Aluminum acetate
Aluminum chloride
Aluminum sulfate
Aniline dyes
  (water-soluble)
Arrowroot
Benzaldehyde
Betanaphthol
Boric acid
Cocoa butter
Cornstarch
Cresol
Dibromfluorescein
Formaldehyde
Geraniol
Gum arabic
Gum karaya
Gum tragacanth
Henna
Lead compounds
Lycopodium
Oil of almond
Oil of bay
Oil of bergamot
Oil of cananga
Oil of cassia

Oil of coriander
Oil of cottonseed
Oil of eucalyptus
Oil of heliotropine
Oil of jasmine
Oil of lemon
Oil of linseed
Oil of Neroli
Oil of orange
Oil of spearmint
Oil of wintergreen
Oxalic acid
Phenol
Phenolformaldehyde
p-Phenylenediamine
Quince seed
Resins
Resorcinol
Rice starch
Rosin
Salicylic acid
Shellac
Sulfonamide resins
Wheat starch
Wool fat
  (crude lanolin)
Zinc chloride
Zinc salicylate
Zinc sulfate

Almay and Ar-Ex do not make as many different products as the lines of other companies, because they have limited themselves to what they can safely use as substitutes for raw materials known as the common allergens. However, these hypo-allergenic products are very attractive, and their manufacturers are adding to these lines all the time. Almay will also, on request from a physician, make up a special product for women with special allergies.

. . .

PSEUDO-HYPO-ALLERGENIC COSMETICS: The legitimate concept of hypo-allergenic products has spawned a host of cosmetics of dubious value, such as the categories below.

Natural cosmetics. These are the most frequently encountered pseudo-hypo-allergenic cosmetics. They are usually based on some vegetable, fruit, or herb, ranging from avocado oil, fresh fruits, herbs, cucumbers, and peaches to more exotic plants. None of these ingredients is of itself usually poisonous, either externally or internally. But before buying any natural cosmetic, remember what really goes into such a product.

The base of these cosmetics is the same as that of most other cosmetics—namely oils, waxes, perfumes, and alcohol. All these chemicals have been shown to cause allergies.

Vegetables, fruits, and herbs are no less allergenic than many of the chemicals commonly found in cosmetics. For example, many people are allergic to strawberries, lemons, or peaches. Adding these "natural" ingredients certainly does not make them less allergy-provoking; only the exclusion of known allergens as described on pages 118–19 can accomplish this. The presence of these plants, or even the addition of soothing herbs like camomile or comfrey root, does not make a product hypo-allergenic.

Organic cosmetics. By legal definition, organic substances are derived from plants or animals that have been raised without the use of hormones, pesticides, or chemical fertilizers. In reality, the label term "organic" is applied to anything the manufacturer wishes. In the field of hypo-allergenic cosmetics, organic usually means the same thing as natural—that is, it contains fruits, vegetables, or herbs. Whatever they are called, these products are no less allergenic than the ingredients from which they are made. Remember, it is really what is left out of a cosmetic that makes it hypo-allergenic, not what is put *into* it.

Doctor-tested cosmetics. This is a loosely used term that means some kind of medical or scientific testing has been done on the product. Such testing could range from a staff of well-trained physicians running a large variety of tests to determine the safety, purity, and allergy potential of the substance to a single experiment done by a chemist on a few laboratory animals. It is not necessarily a guarantee of value.

Dermatologist-tested cosmetics. This term usually indicates a more standardized form of testing. Practicing dermatologists are given samples of products to try on their patients and the results are noted and evaluated by the manufacturer. It is a fairly good indication that the product has been competently evaluated for its allergy potential.

Allergy-tested cosmetics. There are many ways a cosmetic can be evaluated for allergenicity, and this term indicates that in some manner such a test has been run on a particular product. Whether it was a conclusive, thorough experiment or a poorly designed test is known only to the manufacturer.

Doctor-approved cosmetics. This is another loosely worded term often used to indicate that a doctor (either a Ph.D. in biology or chemistry or a medical doctor) has reviewed the formula of a product, and on the basis of current knowledge has decided that this formula is not likely to cause allergies. It is probably the least satisfactory way of testing a product.

Cosmetics designed for sensitive skin. It is not at all clear on what basis these products are better for sensitive skins. They do not list their ingredients, so it is impossible to determine what is in them. The companies that manufacture them do not issue a list of ingredients they exclude to make their products less irritating. Some of these products contain fruits, vegetables, or herbs that they claim soothe the skin. As mentioned before, such products are no less allergenic than regular cosmetics; it is the elimination of sensitizing substances, not the addition of "soothing" ones, that makes a hypo-allergenic cosmetic.

Herbal cosmetics. Herb extracts can and do retain some of their original potency when made into shampoos, face masks, and other cosmetics. Here again, however, the buyer has to be very careful. You must ask yourself—what herbs?

Different herbs have different characteristics and properties, as do different medicines. Some herbs, such as camomile, are very soothing to the skin. Others, such as mint, stimulate blood circulation in the skin. Still other herbs do nothing at all to the skin or hair, while some herbs might produce effects that you would just as well not experience. (See the Glossary for a listing of different herbs used in cosmetic products and descriptions of their effects.)

Medicated cosmetics. Another type of cosmetic is one formulated for acne-troubled skin. These are usually fragrance free, contain some antiseptic or sulfur in their ingredients, and have a low oil content. They are designed primarily to minimize acne problems, but have no value for other kinds of sensitive or splotchy skins.

Although their sulfur and/or antiseptic ingredients are needed to give them their effective anti-acne qualities, most of these same acne-control chemicals are also known to be allergens for many people.

It must be pointed out that the terms above are sometimes used interchangeably and I have given only an ideal breakdown of their characteristics. To really know what you are getting when you buy a hypo-allergenic product you must know what ingredients it contains. Only then will you be able to evaluate the list of ingredients against a list of known allergens and determine if this product has a genuinely lower chance of causing allergy problems.

THOSE WHO NEED HYPO-ALLERGENIC PRODUCTS:

Truly allergic people. They tend to react to common allergens much more readily than others. The likelihood of their reacting to the common sensitizers found in many cosmetics is fairly high. These people have demonstrated repeated allergies to foods, household cleansers, pollens, and to various types of fabrics.

Such allergic women should stick to truly hypo-allergenic products as much as possible. But they should realize that even these hypo-allergenic products can, at times, also cause trouble. Allergic women must make a continuous effort to avoid the worst of the common cosmetic allergens, such as perfumes (which should be sprayed on the clothes, not the skin), bleaching creams, hair dyes, sunscreens containing para-aminobenzoic acid, and depilatories.

When a skin eruption does break out, these women must review everything they use on their skins and try to determine— by elimination of one cosmetic or household cleanser at a time— what is causing the new skin problem.

Occasionally allergy-sensitive people. They have rare but annoying allergies to certain products. They might be allergic, or become so after months or years of use, to Brand X lipstick, and be allergic to nothing else. This allergic reaction causes your lips to become puffy and red every time you use this lipstick.

The allergy could be caused by the perfume in Brand X lipstick. Try switching to a similar color in Brand Y. Same problem? Then it is probably not the perfume. It could be the dye. Try a different color from Brand X. If you suffer a reaction this time, you are probably allergic to something basic to the formulas for all lipsticks of standard manufacturers.

At this point, try a similar lipstick from a good hypo-allergenic line, whose manufacturers have left out some ingredients and added others to decrease the chances of allergic reactions.

However, if you react badly to only this one item—lipstick —or to any other single item, it is not necessary that you switch to the use of hypo-allergenic products exclusively. Take advantage of the wide range of colors and products that standard lines offer. Do not be afraid to use them, and do not think that all hypo-allergenic products are better for everybody's skin. They are better only if you have an allergy.

8 / Outside Influences on the Skin

Sun and the Skin

It is unequivocally true that most people look much better with a suntan. A nice, even, bronze color masks the skin's imperfections, promotes a look of health and well-being, and even implies financial success in terms of "the good life." So the fact that exposure to the sun is just about the worst thing you can do to your skin seems terribly unfair . . . but it is true.

Sun ages the appearance of the skin faster than anything else. It makes oily skin oilier, turns normal skin to dry skin, and encourages acne breakouts in acne-prone skin. However, since most people feel they look better with a tan, there is a way to maximize your tan and minimize the harmful effects of the sun. First it is important to know just how the sun actually harms your skin.

What the Sun Does to Your Skin

Sunlight is made up of many different kinds of rays. The particular rays that change the physical and chemical constitution of the body after exposure to them are known as ultraviolet, or uv, rays. In the process of tanning, the uv rays disrupt certain light-sensitive proteins in the skin. This chemical reaction acts on the skin's blood vessels to produce redness and heat, the first signs of sunburn. The disrupted, light-sensitive proteins also stimulate swelling (edema) of the skin. (You know how swollen and sore your skin feels after eight hours on the beach.) One of the reasons people look so good with the first flush of a sunburn is that the edema puffs out the skin on the face, smoothing out the lines. But, in fact, the edema is a sign of injury similar to a sprain or a bruise. At the same time the skin tries to protect itself by rapidly building a barrier layer of cells as a shield against the sunlight.

Simultaneously, melanocytes (pigment-producing cells) are producing more dark melanin granules, which will give additional protection against the sun. It takes several hours before the granules can be produced and deposited into the cells of the epidermis. (These melanin-enriched cells then travel to the upper layers of the epidermis.) This is why you do not tan immediately in the sun, but only hours or even days later. It takes two to three days before all the melanin produced by a single exposure to sun is well distributed in the top layer of the epidermis.

Once the skin is tanned it seems to need constant exposure to sun, or the "tan" seems to fade. The melanin granules never fade, but the cells that contain them are dying and falling off the skin at a very rapid rate. When the skin is exposed to the sun, the whole process of growth is speeded up to provide a thick outer shield of cells against the sun. This speeded-up state of growth and death does not stop once you get out of the sun. The skin cells are into a big growth cycle that will not stop until most of the effects of the sun have worn off at least several days later. Then, when most of the cells damaged by the sun have passed through the stages of their growth cycle and have flaked off, the skin will go back to its normal growth pattern. By this time your hard-won tan will have disappeared.

The more concentrated or intense the exposure to the sun, the faster the skin tries to protect itself by producing more cells. The more cells it produces, the more cells flake off. The result is that one long (say eight hours) exposure to the sun will promote a great deal of cell growth and subsequent peeling of skin, with rapid loss of tan. On the other hand, eight one-hour exposures will allow the skin to slowly build up a protection against the sun. Since the body was not assaulted so violently, it will not react violently; this new layer of skin will not shed as quickly, and the tan will last much longer.

The ultraviolet rays, unfortunately, do more than cause a tan. They penetrate deeply into the dermis (the skin's lower layer) to disrupt and damage the collagen fibers. In young people, most of this damaged collagen is absorbed by the body and new collagen is formed. But once the body reaches maturity, the ability to produce collagen slows down. This old, damaged collagen will remain and the skin permanently loses its ability to move easily. It can no longer snap back into shape. It sags, making the face baggy and wrinkled.

Sun damage to the collagen is considered the greatest cause of wrinkled skin. A woman of seventy has very wrinkled and baggy skin on her face and hands. But on the parts of the body not exposed to sun, the skin is smooth and unlined.

For all other parts of the body the aging processes seem to be controlled almost entirely by internal changes. But for the skin, aging is strongly influenced by exposure to the sun.

The heat generated by the sun will also dehydrate your skin. You know how rapidly a wet bathing suit dries out in the sun. The same thing is happening to your skin. Dehydrated, water-poor skin is *not* attractive skin.

The epidermis needs water to be attractive, smooth, soft, and supple. Without water, the cells of the top layer of epidermis dry out and crumble; they cannot hold together and they flake off the skin at a rapid rate. The loss of water makes lines and wrinkles seem much deeper. Certainly you have seen how flaky and ugly your skin looks after the first glow of a weekend tan wears off. This unattractive appearance is mostly caused by the severe dehydration of your skin.

Finally, the sun causes skin cancer. It has been shown that states with more sunshine, such as Arizona and Texas, have ten to fifteen times as much skin cancer as states such as Massachusetts or Illinois, which have far fewer sunny days. Furthermore, skin cancer rarely appears in areas of the body not exposed to sunlight.

You can cheat on some things with the sun. You can stop dehydration with oils. You can start having face lifts at thirty-five to pick up the slack tissue caused by shattered collagen fibers. But you cannot cheat on skin cancer. It is almost always disfiguring, because the doctors have to remove great amounts of skin, along with cancerous growths.

. . .

How to Deal with the Sun

The first defense against the sun is a good commercial sunscreen preparation. Sunscreens, both creams and lotions, act by two principles.

Some sunscreens provide a total covering that will exclude all sun rays. The other class of preparations contains a substance that will exclude only the ultraviolet rays, not allowing them to penetrate the skin.

The first of the two principal forms of sunscreen is used when you want *total* protection from the sun. This sunscreen is a thick white paste often made with zinc oxide. It is used by lifeguards and swimmers, most often to cover the nose and lips. It is often wise to use such a sunscreen around the eyes, where the skin is very thin and very susceptible to sunburn.

The second type of sunscreen has the ability to resist some or most of the ultraviolet rays. The simplest form of this type of sunscreen is plain oil. Sesame seed oil is best for this form of protection. It resists 30 percent of the ultraviolet rays. It is available at health food stores at about 10 cents an ounce. Coconut oil, peanut oil, olive oil, and cottonseed oil resist about 20 percent of the uv rays. Mineral oil does not resist any of the sun's rays. This fact is particularly interesting since many people use baby oil, which contains mostly mineral oil, as a suntan lotion. In addition, mineral oil dissolves sebum, the secretion of the oil glands, which is especially needed during sunbathing in order to slow down the evaporation of water from the skin.

A more complete sunscreen than any of these is obtained when certain chemicals are added to vegetable oil. There are many of these additives, but the best of them is para-aminobenzoic acid (PABA for short). Two commercial products that contain PABA are SKOLEX and SKOL by Williams. The next best sunscreen additives are the *salicylate compounds*. These ingredients prevent the uv rays from hitting the skin. The degree to which they work depends on their concentration in the sunscreen.

PABA and salicylates are both active ingredients and must be listed on the label. If a suntan product does not list any ingredients, it is nothing more than a mixture of oils, waxes, and emulsifiers, and thus gives relatively scant protection against the sun.

Sunscreens come in many forms: oils, lotions, creams, and

aerosols. For every type of skin other than oily or acned skin, the oilier the lotion, the better its protection. This means that it contains fewer emulsifiers, such as soap, which dehydrate the skin.

Oily lotions are sticky to use and can stain your bathing suit, so be careful when you put on such a product. It's a good idea to use a small natural sponge instead of your fingers to spread it on your body. Wipe your hands well after using it.

Every suntan product must be reapplied every three hours. Evaporation, perspiration, and swimming will wash off the sunscreen and render the skin vulnerable once again to the sun.

How the Skin Can Protect Itself

The next layer of defense against the sun is the skin itself. As you know, the ultraviolet rays stimulate the skin to produce more cells, which form a thicker layer of skin. If these cells are produced too rapidly, the skin sheds the new layer quickly.

The idea is to produce enough cells to form additional protection against the sun without stimulating rapid sloughing off of the cells. This is done by small exposures to the sun. Each exposure to the sun causes the skin to grow just a bit thicker. Little by little a protective barrier is formed and the skin can take more sun with less damage to collagen fibers and other tissues deep in the skin. The slow building up of the protective layer discourages the rapid loss of the top layers, and as a result the tan remains for a longer time. This is why you should start with small doses of sun.

SOME DO'S AND DON'T'S OF SUNTANNING

1. Start with a fifteen-minute exposure. Then, each day, add another fifteen minutes. Never sit directly in the sun longer than two hours. You will not get any better tan; in fact, you will lose it more rapidly.

The protective coating principle of slow sun exposure also pertains to melanin production—the process responsible for giving your skin a tan color. Melanin production is the body's attempt to put up a dark screen against the sun. You must give your body a chance to produce and distribute its melanin products. This melanin will prevent or diminish the ultraviolet rays from going deep into the dermis, where the collagen fibers are located.

2. The sun's burning rays are at their strongest between eleven a.m. and two p.m. Avoid the sun as much as possible during these hours. Get all your sunning done in the early morning or the late afternoon.

3. Limit your total yearly sunbathing to no more than thirty days.

4. Ultraviolet rays are extremely penetrating. You can sustain changes to your collagen fibers from the light that comes through a window, even on a cloudy day.

5. Try alternatives to the sun. Artificial tanning lotions are good for promoting a healthy bronze look without the problems of a natural tan. But they do not provide any protection against the sun. They do not turn the skin brown by stimulating melanin production, but by the action of a chemical commonly known as D.H.A., which causes superficial browning of the skin when it combines with the free amino acids in the top layer of the epidermis. Since this layer is the very topmost layer and is constantly being shed, the artificial tan does not last very long, usually no more than a week. To avoid an orange cast to the skin, do not apply it more frequently than every two weeks to be on the safe side. Nevertheless, artificial tanners have been shown to be quite safe for the skin. Very few allergic reactions have been reported, and it is definitely not carcinogenic (as are the sun's rays). One commonly found product of this type is Q.T. TANNING OIL or LOTION by Coppertone.

When You Get Out of the Sun

After you get out of the sun, wash your face and body with mild soap and water to remove the accumulated oil, sweat, and suntan oil. If, despite all these warnings, you get too much sun, do not slather your body with oils. They will keep all the heat in your skin and increase the damage produced by the burn. You should first get into a tepid tub into which you've dissolved two cups of laundry starch (like LINIT) or oatmeal. Sit in the tub for twenty minutes. The tepid water and starch will reduce the inflammation and redness of the burn. After twenty minutes wash your skin gently with a mild bland soap.

Once you have finished your bath, dry yourself off gently. Smooth on a small amount of a soothing cream like VITAMIN A AND D OINTMENT by White or one of the creams rich in allantoin (a healing agent that helps the damaged skin return to normal).

Even after bathing do not be too liberal with soothing cream; it will simply keep the heat in.

Many people think that if they pour creams and lotions on their skin it will not flake off; unfortunately, oiling simply lets the skin regain a good moisture level. The moisture speeds the normalization of the skin after a burn. But if skin has had too much sun at one time, the excess cells that grew to protect the skin have to flake off and oil won't stop them from doing so. If you have oily skin, it's much better not to use any oil at all.

Try to make a little tan go a long way. Do not use all your tanning days at once. Take the sun for a maximum of three or four days. Then nurse the resulting tan along with artificial tanners and cosmetic bronzes. With this method your tan can last about two weeks for every three to four days of exposure to the sun. With a three-day suntan stretched out to last for two weeks your thirty days of allowed sun time will give you a nice bronze glow for five months out of the year.

Smoking, Alcohol, Drugs— And Your Skin

Smoking, heavy drinking, and drugs can destroy your appearance as well as your life.

The Skin and Smoking

Besides increasing your chances for heart disease, emphysema, and lung cancer, smoking has been shown to prematurely age and wrinkle skin. Dr. Harry W. Daniell of Redding, California, recently published the results of a clinical study in which he compared the skin of smoking and nonsmoking individuals. He found that in every age group the individuals who smoked heavily had much more yellowed and wrinkled skin than nonsmokers. Look at the photographs below:

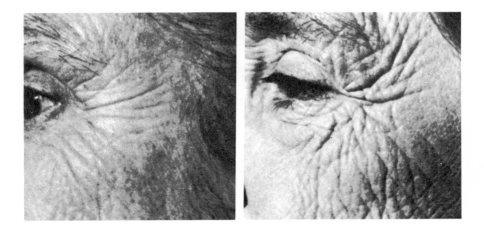

Dr. Daniell feels that this accelerated aging is due to the presence of nicotine in tobacco. Nicotine causes the small blood vessels in the skin to contract, and thereby decrease the skin's circulation. The slower the circulation, the less blood can flow through the skin's blood vessels. Since the healthy pink coloration of the skin is due in large part to the color of the blood circulating under the skin's surface, less blood circulation means less of this pink color; thus the skin looks yellow and sallow.

If you smoke, try these treatments once or twice weekly to stimulate the circulation. These treatments will not stop the damage smoking causes to your skin, but it might look a little better. Remember that the best treatment is to stop smoking!

A PROGRAM OF CARE FOR SMOKER'S SKIN

NORMAL/DRY SKIN

1. Wash with a water-soluble cream.

2. Steam your face with a sauna for ten to fifteen minutes.

3. Use a gel mask with mint or yeast (MINT MASQUE by Revlon is such a product).

OILY SKIN

1. Wash with soap and water.

2. Steam your face with a sauna for ten to fifteen minutes, or use a hot-towel treatment for the same length of time.

3. Use a clay mask with a mint or yeast additive.

The Skin and Alcohol

Light drinking is not harmful to the skin. A little wine, or one martini, dilates the blood vessels and in fact creates a nice healthy blush in the skin. Moderate to heavy drinking is another story. The dilating effect alcohol has on the blood vessels can, after a period of time, cause tiny blood vessels to burst. These are seen as small red lines on the face and body. They can ruin an otherwise attractive complexion.

Alcohol robs the skin of water. You know how dry and thirsty your mouth feels the morning after. Well, your skin is dry and thirsty also. The alcohol leaches water out of the tissues, making normal or dry skin flaky and dull. It is very important to try to replace the water after drinking a great deal of alcohol. Drink plenty of fluids (water, fruit juice, tea, or coffee), then try this water-replenishment treatment for the skin.

A PROGRAM OF CARE FOR DRINKER'S SKIN

NORMAL/DRY SKIN

1. Wash your face with a water-soluble cream.

2. Steam your face with a sauna for ten minutes.

3. Rinse about ten or fifteen times with cool water.

4. Apply a generous amount of N.M.F. cream and let it soak into the skin.

OILY SKIN

1. Wash with a mild soap, like DOVE. Do not use your regular oily skin soap.

2. Steam your face with a sauna for ten minutes.

3. Rinse ten to fifteen times with cool water.

4. Put on a gel mask, to create a watertight shield and let the skin build up a supply of water.

5. Leave the mask on for thirty minutes, rinse your face again with cool water.

6. Do not use any oil or "moisturizer." The oil will merely make an oily skin oilier.

The Skin and Drugs

There are so many beauty problems one has no control over —overactive glands, dry skin, or thin hair. The skin problems due to drugs, however, are all self-inflicted and unnecessary. Virtually all the "abused" drugs affect the skin's appearance.

Amyl nitrites, commonly called "sniffers" or "poppers," interfere with the body's ability to obtain oxygen. The skin actually turns blue for a short time. Not only does the skin look awful, but the lack of oxygen also slows down cell growth and in this way prematurely ages the skin.

Glue sniffing irritates the skin around the nose so much that it may peel off, leaving a large oozing area on the upper lip.

Dr. Irwin Lubowe, a noted New York dermatologist, has found that habitual use of marijuana can cause hair loss and aggravate acne if it is already present. Marijuana can also cause "red-eye" (conjunctivitis), as well as allergic reactions like hives or asthma.

Tranquilizers and "downers" have been known to cause an allergic rash or widespread shedding of the skin.

Barbiturates can cause similar reactions, as well as causing large "barbiturate blisters" around the mouth and at pressure points of the body, such as the ankles or the hips.

Amphetamines, or "uppers," or "speed," can cause allergic reactions such as rashes or asthma attacks. Even low doses of these drugs make the mouth and lips very dry. People who use them are always licking their lips, which may cause severe chapping and sores of the mouth and lips.

Heroin can totally wreck your appearance. The areas in which drugs are injected become scarred, veins are stopped up with blood clots; ulcers, infections, blisters, and abscesses can develop. In addition, addicts tend to develop dark circles under their eyes. Their skin usually loses its elasticity at an early age. Perhaps most important, one's favorable self-image disappears, and with this loss of self-identity there is also the loss of all the basic grooming and body maintenance routines we take for granted. A woman addict will frequently look much older than her actual age.

There are no real remedies to the problems that drugs cause to your skin, your body, and your whole person. The results of their use are chronic, and all too often devastating.

9 / Special Problems of the Skin

Excess Hair

Excess hair on the face and body is one of the most distressing beauty problems that can plague a woman. It is unfortunately one of the most difficult ones to cope with successfully. The problem can range from a slightly heavy growth of hair on the upper lip to a full facial beard. Most popular discussions of this problem do not go into the various conditions that cause unwanted hair, but concentrate on analyzing and evaluating the pro's and con's of shaving depilatories, waxing, and electrolysis. Many conditions that cause unwanted hair to grow can be corrected, however, and the hair will disappear after treatment of the underlying medical problem.

What Constitutes Excess Hair

For a woman the presence of excess hair on her face is a very sensitive issue. Because there are serious medical conditions that can cause excess hair, or *hirsutism*, it is important to understand what constitutes an abnormal growth of hair and what constitutes merely a normal variation of the female growth pattern.

The most common spot for a woman to grow visible facial hair is her upper lip. If this area is the only part of the face where there is a noticeable growth of hair, if the cheeks and chin area seem smooth and hairless, the chances are that this condition is within a normal range of facial hair growth. The odds that it is normal are increased if the mustache can be made almost invisible by local bleaching. This kind of hair growth will also respond fairly well to removal by electrolysis.

However, mild to heavy growth on the upper lip, the sides of the face, and on the chin points to more than a normal variation of hair growth, and for most women suggests that an underlying problem might be causing excess hair to grow.

How Body and Facial Hair Grows

From head to foot there are very few areas of the body where hair cannot grow heavily. Fortunately, nature smiles on the average woman and this growth of hair is normally minimal or invisible on the face and body.

The biological machinery for growing the hair is called the hair follicle. This is a U-shaped sac, or depression, in the skin. It contains a hair root shaped like a bulb as well as an oil and sweat gland. The opening through which the hair grows is the same opening through which oil and perspiration reach the skin's surface (see Diagram 3, page 7).

Under normal circumstances, the hair follicle produces a very fine, almost invisible hair. In many follicles, no hair is actually growing, but the ability to produce a hair still exists. In certain situations, however, the hair follicle receives the wrong signal from the body. Instead of producing fine, thin hair, it grows a thick, coarse hair that is quite apparent on the skin's surface.

The rate and kind of hair growth in the follicle are controlled primarily by the hormones produced by the ovaries and adrenal glands. These in turn are governed by the hormones of the pituitary gland, the tiny "master" gland at the base of the brain. A problem affecting the normal activity of any of these three glands can cause a prominent increase in the amount of unwanted hair.

Hirsutism and the Ovaries

A common cause of hirsutism is a malfunction of the ovaries. The ovary produces three main groups of hormones—estrogens, progesterones, and androgens. The amount of hormones that this gland produces has a profound effect on the manifestation of most female characteristics: the size of the breasts, the regularity of the menstrual period, the growth pattern of hair on the face and body, weight, and amount of oil produced on the skin and scalp.

When the ovaries produce abnormal amounts of any or all of these three hormones the results can be infertility, oily skin and hair, and, of course, excess hair.

The most frequent problems that cause the ovaries to malfunction are cysts and tumors. The presence of these abnormal growths on the ovaries causes them to produce abnormal amounts of hormones.

The diagnosis of ovarian cysts is made by a doctor's physical examination, a careful analysis of your medical history, as well as blood and urine examinations. When the ovary has many cysts, these may possibly be felt during an internal examination.

Your medical history is important because, in addition to an excess amount of facial hair, a woman with *polycystic* (many cysts) ovaries will complain of irregular menses, infertility, acne, and overweight.

What causes the ovaries to form cysts is not yet known. The symptoms usually appear in the eighteen to thirty-five age group. There are two different forms of treatment, surgical and medical.

With the surgical approach, a small wedge is cut out of the ovary. For reasons not really understood this seems to make the ovary function better. The menses become regular, and many women are then able to conceive. The growth of new hair is stopped, but the existing hairs usually do not fall out. These, however, can be removed by electrolysis.

The medical approach consists in giving the body relatively high doses of estrogens and progesterones. These hormones normally regulate the menstrual periods, reduce the hair's oiliness, clear up acne, discourage the growth of new and unwanted hair on the face and body. Existing hair will fall out and will not grow in again.

Ovarian tumors may produce many of the signs and symptoms described for the condition of polycystic ovaries—acne, irregular periods, and excess hair. But when tumors are present, the hair growth is very severe, with a thick growth of hair on the chin, the cheeks, the upper lip, around the breasts, and on the stomach and back. In addition, a deepening of the voice and a decrease in breast size may occur. During an internal examination by your doctor, the tumor may be felt on the ovary.

Unlike polycystic ovaries, whose symptoms slowly appear between the ages of eighteen to thirty-five, an ovarian tumor usually develops rapidly and at any age.

Therapy consists of removal of the tumor. In this case, supplemental hormones may be necessary to replace those normally produced by the healthy ovary. After successful surgery, all signs of the tumor may disappear. The hair, oiliness, and acne may vanish and the breasts may return to their normal size. Not all ovarian tumors produce these problems, but since many of them do result in excess hair, they are included as a group in this chapter.

Hirsutism and the Adrenal and Pituitary Glands

The adrenal glands are located in the abdomen, on top of each kidney. They secrete three major types of hormones: cortisone (and its close relatives), androgens, and aldosterone. *Cortisone* has many functions in the body and affects virtually every other gland and part of the body. *Androgens* (the "male" sex hormones) in a woman are necessary for proper bone development; they regulate the secretion of oil produced by the skin's oil glands; and they play a major role in determining sexual characteristics. Androgens are, in fact, the most important hormone of the adrenal glands when considering problems of excess hair. It is the level of androgens in the body that directly controls the activity of the hair follicles. The greater the amount of androgen, the more hair will grow. *Aldosterone*, which regulates salt levels in the body, is the third hormone produced by the adrenal glands, but it does not affect hair growth.

Any problem that affects the adrenal glands may affect the amount of any or all of these hormones. For example, an adrenal tumor can cause a huge increase in the amount of cortisone and androgens. This may cause obesity, acne, changes in bone structure, and increased growth of facial and body hair. The diagnosis is made on the basis of a doctor's physical examination, specific blood and urine tests, and sometimes X-rays.

Treatment consists, whenever possible, in the removal of the tumor. After successful surgery, most of the symptoms that resulted from the hormonal imbalance will completely disappear.

Any hair that may not fall out can be removed at this time by electrolysis.

Malfunction of the adrenal glands may occur without a tumor being present. For example, at the time of puberty, the adrenal glands may begin producing too much hormone. For some unknown reason, glandular signals become crossed and excess amounts of androgen and/or cortisone are produced. Characteristically, girls with the problem have irregular menstrual periods, perhaps only once or twice a year, underdeveloped breasts, and excessive facial hair.

Treatment usually consists of continued administration of prednisone (an artificial form of cortisone), which calms down the overactive adrenal gland and coaxes it to produce the right amount of hormones. After several years of this therapy, the excess facial hair disappears, breast development becomes normal, and periods become regular.

A tumor of the pituitary (master) gland can influence a normal adrenal gland to produce too much hormone, causing problems similar to those produced by an adrenal tumor. Increasing facial hair, obesity, and acne may be prominent features. Treatment usually involves radiation therapy of the pituitary.

Both adrenal and pituitary tumors can occur at any age and the effects will be quite noticeable, so that early medical advice is sought.

These problems with the adrenal and pituitary glands account for about 15 percent of women with excess hair.

Other Causes of Hirsutism

So far the causes underlying an estimated 50 percent of the cases of excess hair have been discussed. In each of these circumstances a specific problem has been found that causes the glands to malfunction, producing abnormal amounts of hormones, and thereby causing excess hair growth.

In the remaining 50 percent of women who suffer from excess hair, diagnosis of a specific cause has not been possible. None of the usual causes were found: no major disease in any of the hormone-producing glands, no tumors, no gross malformations of the glands, and no cysts.

It seems that certain ethnic groups (e.g., Jews, Italians, and other Mediterranean people) are more naturally hairy than other groups (e.g., the Scandinavians and Orientals). At the same time, these people frequently have dark hair that can appear prominent on the face even when the amount is not excessive.

Sometimes excess facial hair growth seems to run in families and could be the result of an inherited genetic factor.

Some endocrinologists feel that in certain women, excess hair is due to an increased sensitivity to the levels of androgens on the part of the hair follicles. These women are putting out normal amounts of hormones, yet for some unknown reason, this triggers a follicle to grow stiff, dark hairs.

In cases where no underlying cause can be found, doctors will usually offer cosmetic therapy of electrolysis or waxing (pages 145 and 146). In severe cases, however, a doctor might prescribe a course of cortisone therapy, in hopes of suppressing adrenal androgen production. It has been found that when the adrenal gland is overproductive, the presence of extra cortisone slows it down. This slowing down of the gland affects, in particular, those cells in the gland producing unwanted androgens.

The cortisone stops the growth of new hair, and encourages the hair already growing to fall out. Any stubborn hair can be easily removed by electrolysis with no fears that new hairs will crop up in other areas, as sometimes happens when the underlying condition is not cleared up and electrolysis is used.

About 60 percent of women start to grow facial hair after their menopause. This is due to widespread hormonal changes in the body that go along with menopause. This kind of hirsutism may sometimes be controlled by estrogen therapy commonly used to treat many of the other symptoms of menopause. In theory, this therapy normalizes the hormone balance in the body and the growth of unwanted hair should stop. Much of the postmenopausal hair that has grown in will fall out. Some, however, usually remains and has to be removed by electrolysis or other hair-removal methods.

One final point should be kept in mind. Many women feel that cold creams and estrogen creams produce excess hair on the face. This simply is not so. Women often start using these creams in their late forties, when excess facial hair first becomes apparent. These two events are only coincidental. The hormone changes in a woman's body that make her skin dry and necessitate the use of moisturizers also cause the growth of unwanted facial hair.

Hair Removal

ELECTROLYSIS: Electrolysis works by passing an electric current through an electric needle into the hair follicle to destroy the hair root bulb. It is not painful, but it can be expensive and time-consuming. The electric needle has to reach the hair bulb at exactly the right angle in order to destroy it. If it does not, the hair will grow back. Usually even a skilled electrolysis operator has to attack a hair root several times before it stops producing hairs. Despite these drawbacks, electrolysis can permanently remove hair from small areas. However, it should never be undertaken until a thorough physical examination has been performed by your doctor to determine whether there is any underlying cause to the hair growth you wish removed. If there is and it is not treated, no matter how much hair is removed, new hair will continue to spring up in nearby follicles. Under these circumstances electrolysis is an unending and futile process.

SHAVING: Shaving with a razor cuts the hair off at the skin level. It does a very adequate, albeit temporary, job of hair removal. It is an excellent method for removing a light growth of hair from legs and underarms. While many women shave the hair from these parts of the body they understandably balk at the thought of shaving hair from the face.

CHEMICAL DEPILATORIES: These are products made up of thioglycolic acid, chalk, wax, and water. The thioglycolic acid breaks the bonds of the hair, weakening the hair enough so that it can be broken off and scraped away. The hair comes off at the skin level or slightly below.

While depilatories take off hair easily, and the hairs do not grow back as rapidly as after shaving there are, nevertheless, several drawbacks to using depilatories. The thioglycolic acid is an extremely caustic chemical and one to which many people develop an allergy.

Contrary to popular belief, shaving and depilatories do *not.*

increase the growth of hair. What actually happens is that the hair that grows in after the original hair has been removed looks coarser and thicker. Normally the hair shaft tapers to a point, which is much narrower than the rest of the shaft. When you shave a hair you cut it off at the skin level, which is somewhere in the middle of the hair shaft. The new tip of the shaved hair is now of the same thickness as the rest of the hair, giving the appearance that coarser and more abundant hair is growing.

WAXING: Hot wax is poured on the skin, left to dry, then peeled off, thus removing the hair and its root. It will take from three to six weeks for a waxed hair to grow back. This is not a permanent form of hair removal, since waxing does not destroy the hair bulb, where the hair is originally formed. However, after waxing, many of the hair bulbs are damaged and *no longer produce hair.* Because waxing pulls out the whole hair, the new hair grows in with a point and is neither stubby nor thick. This is the most efficient way of removing hair from a large area, such as the sides of the face.

A very successful method of hair removal for the face would combine both waxing and electrolysis: waxing for the sides of the face, and electrolysis for the upper lip. Both techniques should be performed by professionals. Electrolysis should be done by licensed electrolysis operators. Many dermatologists will often know good ones to refer you to. Waxing is done by cosmetologists and beauticians. Home electrolysis and hot wax kits are available, but I would advise against them; hair removal is tricky and should be done by someone who has proper training and experience.

X-RAYS: In past years, X-rays were used to remove excess facial hair. The rays killed the hair-growing cells and did decrease the hair. But a few years after this treatment, some women who had this treatment developed skin cancer. Because of this danger, X-rays have been abandoned by doctors for the treatment of cosmetic problems.

BLEACHING: Bleaching the hair is a good way of dealing with a very light growth of dark hair. The bleach, a combination of peroxide, ammonia, and soap flakes, is applied to the desired area of the skin. It is left on for five minutes and then rinsed off. This technique lightens the hair so that it blends in better with the skin. It is only effective where there is a small amount of unwanted hair. When a great deal of unwanted hair is present the end result of bleaching will be a noticeable blond or reddish-blond mustache.

BLEACHING TECHNIQUE

BLEACH FORMULA

2 tablespoons twenty-volume peroxide, 6 percent (available from the druggist)

15 drops ammonia

1 tablespoon pure soap flakes (such as Ivory Snow)

Mix together.

BLEACHING PROCEDURE

1. Apply mixture to face with cotton swab.

2. Leave on for thirty minutes.

3. Rinse off with cool water.

4. If area is irritated (as sometimes happens), pat on a soothing lotion such as a vitamin A and D preparation.

Enlarged Pores

The pore is the small hole through which oil secreted by the sebaceous glands flows to the skin's surface. This is also the opening through which the hair grows. Usually this pore is invisible to the eye, but under certain circumstances it becomes enlarged and unsightly.

There are three very different causes of enlarged pores, and all three can be managed or minimized. Once the pore is enlarged, however, it can never truly be reduced. Nevertheless, there is a variety of treatments that can make the pore appear smaller.

Enlarged Pores and Oily Skin

Oily skin is very prone to the problem of large pores. If the glands secrete too much oil, the oil gets blocked up on the way to the surface of the skin. The excess oil stretches the pore opening, which creates an enlarged pore. Limiting oil production is the basis for the control of this type of large pore. Follow the complete program for the care of oily skin on pages 46–50 and, in addition, once or twice a week try this treatment, which will make the pores seem smaller temporarily:

A TREATMENT FOR ENLARGED PORES AND OILY SKIN

1. Cleanse your face thoroughly.

2. Use a sauna for ten to fifteen minutes.

3. Soak several large (4-inch) squares of cotton in an astringent, and wring them out.

4. Lie down and apply the cotton squares to the forehead, chin, cheeks, and nose areas.

5. Remove the astringent pads and let the face dry.

6. Apply foundation and other makeup.

Astringent products that make pores seem smaller all act on the same principle—they cause a slight edema (puffiness) around the pore. The tissue swells up and obstructs the pore opening from sight. See Diagram 20.

Diagram 20.

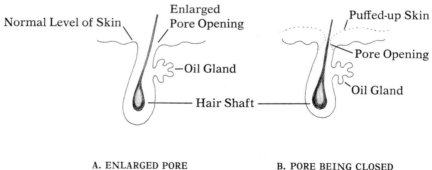

A. ENLARGED PORE   B. PORE BEING CLOSED BY ASTRINGENT

Enlarged Pores and Dry Skin

Dry or wrinkled skin is also prone to develop enlarged pores. Remember, this kind of skin has lost its resiliency and bounce and has started to sag. This sagging effect also occurs around the pores. The skin falls away from the pores, making them seem larger and more prominent. The best way to prevent this kind of enlarged pore is to follow a program of skin care that encourages good skin tone, such as those described on pages 37–41 and 42–4. Choose the one that suits your skin type best. Even if you already have dry skin and enlarged pores, a careful program of skin care will slow down the loosening of the skin and will add tone and smoothness. Here is a special program for additional aid:

A TREATMENT FOR ENLARGED PORES AND DRY SKIN

1. Cleanse the skin with a washable cream.

2. Make up a lotion consisting of ¼ teaspoon of powdered alum (available in the supermarket) to three tablespoonfuls of a thin creamy lotion like LUBRIDERM or NIVEA.

3. Cut out several large squares of cotton, wet them in water, then saturate them with the alum lotion.

4. Lie down, put the saturated cotton squares on the forehead, cheeks, chin, and the bridge of your nose and let them remain for fifteen to twenty minutes.

5. Remove the cotton pads, and wipe off the excess cream.

6. Apply makeup.

The results of this beauty treatment will last only a few hours. Thereafter the edema (swelling) around the pores will decrease and the pores will look large once again.

Large "Pores" and Cystic Acne

Large pores that remain after severe or cystic acne are actually scars formed in the skin as a result of the chronic inflammation of these eruptions. These are not really stretched pores, but are what are descriptively called "ice pick" scars. These scars remain when the skin is affected by large, deep acne pustules. These local areas of infection lead to an erosion of the follicles and the pores. The damage is so deep and complete that regular astringent pore treatments will not make these holes seem smaller. Dermabrasion is the only way to improve the appearance of this kind of skin (see page 64). After dermabrasion, the astringent pore treatment for oily skin will benefit this skin.

Sallow Skin

Until the turn of the century the ultimate in skin beauty was always the pale-white, fragile, porcelain look. This pallid ideal dominated many societies for thousands of years.

The wealthy women of Imperial Rome, in their efforts to achieve the fashionable pale look, used a lead-based face powder, achieving a genuine pallor, since it caused many of them to die from lead poisoning!

The women of Western civilization, from medieval times to the turn of the present century, sought the image of pale, white skin. "Elaine the fair . . . Elaine, the lily maid of Astolat" was celebrated by Tennyson. All the fashionable ladies in Gainsborough's portraits boasted the white-skinned look that was so highly regarded and sought after.

Women went to great lengths to achieve and maintain this absolutely white complexion, using arsenic washes and other dangerous beauty aids. They avoided the sun religiously, never going out without a large hat when the sun shone. During the seventeenth century, the sun parasol made its debut in Europe, and found centuries of use and favor in the hands of European and American women who regularly used liberal applications of white powder to cover their skin and make it seem whiter.

In *Gigi*, Colette's novel of the French courtesans, the grand-aunt, a great courtesan in her time, is appalled to find what she fears is the beginning of a freckle on Gigi's nose. To the grandaunt, this is a blight on the complexion. Little did the courtesans and the women of fashion of Gigi's youth know that the pale skin ideal was even then on its way out.

A few years later, Mademoiselle Coco Chanel returned from a few weeks at Deauville with a light suntan and a rosy glow. In a matter of weeks, all Paris was talking about the way she looked. Other women decided to copy her, and the porcelain, pale complexion lost its magic as the major criterion of beauty. In its place came the ideal of a warm, rich, natural color that still prevails today. Now women work just as hard to have a pink, rosy complexion as they formerly strove to achieve the dead-white look.

Success in controlling your skin color is a matter of knowing how the skin forms its natural pigmentation, and what makes one person ruddy, while another has an olive-toned skin, and a third is copper-complexioned.

What Gives Skin Its Colors

There are three important pigments that lend color to the skin: melanin, which gives skin its brown tones; carotene, which imparts the yellow skin tones; and hemoglobin, the red pigment in the blood, which gives skin its pink and red hues.

These three pigments act together to produce the skin's ultimate color on the same principle that causes you to see green when you look at a blue light through a yellow filter. Our skin color is, actually, a blend of various pigmentations of differing colors. The three pigments—melanin, carotene, and hemoglobin— join one another to produce our flesh tones. But, while all three pigments contribute to the skin's appearance, the rosy, pretty color of beautiful skin is dependent primarily on the red pigment, hemoglobin. Lack of what we now describe as good healthy color is, usually, related to either low hemoglobin levels in the blood or the impaired circulation of blood in the skin.

The Causes of Pallid Skin

There are four basic causes of pallid skin: anemia, exhaustion or illness, poor blood circulation, and thick skin.

ANEMIA: The lack of red blood corpuscles in the blood is a major cause of pale skin. The red corpuscles are the hemoglobin-carrying cells of the blood. There are many types of anemia, from many different causes, and the study and treatment of these disorders form the bulk of the work of the medical subspecialty of hematology.

In the young, premenopausal woman, anemia is fairly common, and is due most often to the regular loss of blood during each menstrual period. Hematologists estimate that in the United States 5 percent of adult women and even greater percentages of adolescent girls have this type of anemia.

Such anemia is usually a minor problem, and can readily be controlled by increasing the amount of iron-rich foods in the diet.

As you can see from the table below, listing the amounts of iron contained in average servings of various common foodstuffs, there is no shortage of iron-rich foods to suit nearly every taste.

IRON CONTENT OF SOME COMMON FOODS

FOOD	MILLIGRAMS OF IRON
1 egg	1.1
3 oz. red meat	2.9
3 oz. lamb	1.0
3 oz. chicken	1.4
3 oz. pork	2.7
3 oz. canned clams	3.5
1 cup of raw oysters	13.0
3 oz. shrimp, cooked	2.6
3 oz. sardines	2.5
1 cup of cow peas, cooked	3.2
1 cup of beet greens, cooked	2.8
1 cup of dandelion greens, cooked	3.2
1 head of Boston lettuce	4.4
1 cup of peas, cooked	2.9
1 cup of spinach, cooked	4.0
1 cup of pitted dates	5.3
1 cup of prune juice	10.5
1 cup of bran flakes	12.3
1 slice of white bread (enriched)	0.6
1 cup of walnuts	7.6
1 cup of asparagus, cooked*	4.1
1 cup of asparagus, drained	0.9

*Plus the cooking liquid, as most of the iron is in this liquid.

There is no absolute amount of iron required at any age for the average woman, but doctors generally agree that a dietary intake of between fifteen and twenty milligrams of dietary iron per day is an adequate supply of this vital mineral. In certain instances, when there is a particularly heavy menstrual flow, or during pregnancy, a doctor might recommend supplementing the diet with iron pills. While this might seem to be more convenient than watching the iron content in your foods, it has two drawbacks. The iron in the pills is not as well absorbed by your body as is the iron found naturally in foods. Iron pills, in addition, may be unpleasant to take; they may be constipating and may upset your stomach. If you do not absolutely need them, it is much better to get your iron from meats, vegetables, and whole grains than from pills.

EXHAUSTION AND ILLNESS: These cause a normally pink and healthy complexion to become pale and sallow. When the body is in a stress situation, some of the blood is shunted from the skin to more important organs and functions necessary for health. When the stress or the illness is overcome, the circulation returns to its normal state. In the meantime, the program of care for pale skin caused by poor circulation can be followed to give the skin a temporary boost in color. Rest, relaxation, and treatment of any illness are, of course, the most important ways of dealing with this cause of pale skin.

POOR BLOOD CIRCULATION: This can also cause pale skin color. The blood may contain plenty of hemoglobin, but if it moves slowly and sluggishly through the blood vessels, or if the blood vessels are themselves damaged, the skin's color will be paler than if the blood were adequately circulated.

After fifty the blood circulation slows down in all parts of the body. This causes many physical changes, including a pale or sallow complexion. The best way to handle this problem is by using masks and lotions that contain rubefactants. These substances stimulate blood circulation in the skin and can give your face a temporarily rosy complexion.

THICK SKIN: A final cause of pale color is surprising. The blood can be red and healthy, the circulation can be excellent, but *the skin itself may be so thick* that the bright red color of the blood cannot show through enough to give a rosy tone to it.

Signs of thick skin include oiliness, good tanning capacity, and no freckles. Many people of southern European descent or origin have this type of thick skin. It is a relatively healthy type of skin to have, and very attractive except for its often sallow color.

This type of skin must be kept super clean to avoid any additional thickness caused by dead cells building up on the surface of the skin. A circulation-stimulating mask should be used frequently, at least three times a week.

It is quite possible to have all the causes of pallid skin simultaneously. For example, a middle-aged woman of Italian descent who complains of chronic fatigue may have all the causes of pallor. She may benefit from more iron and a good rest, as well as from the beauty program for thick skin.

Here is a safe, easy, and usually successful program to give this kind of skin a temporary boost in circulation, usually lasting several hours:

A PROGRAM OF CARE FOR SALLOW SKIN

1. Cleanse with a mild soap or a washable cream.
2. Steam the face with a sauna.
3. Rinse with cool water.
4. Apply a mask containing a mint or a yeast additive. Both of these are rubefactants, and temporarily stimulate the superficial blood circulation of the face.
5. Let the mask dry and set.
6. Rinse mask off.
7. Pat your skin briskly with an astringent.

Massage can also stimulate the blood circulation, but it tends to damage the skin and cause wrinkles (see page 83).

Circulation-stimulating masks create none of these massage problems. They make the face rosier, and are also inexpensive and easy to use. They can be applied often without subjecting the skin to any danger.

Part Two / The Eyes

10 / Beauty Problems of the Eyes and Eye Area

The eyes and the eye area are extremely sensitive to physical changes both inside the body and in the environment. They can become bloodshot, teary, puffy, and develop dark circles. The skin around the eyes has a tendency to form lines and become baggy. But while the eyes may be one of the most delicate parts of the body, their beauty problems are frequently easy to solve.

The Eyes

Bloodshot Eyes

The eyes are covered with a thin colorless membrane that contains many tiny blood vessels. When the eyes are normal, these blood vessels are invisible. But when the eyes are irritated by allergies, too much reading, pollution, lack of sleep, or cigarette smoke, the blood vessels expand and fill up with an increased supply of blood, which makes them appear as thin red lines in the eyes.

Immediate treatment consists of washing out the eyes with an isotonic solution. This is simply a liquid that has the same concentration of salts as normally found in the eye tissues; if such a washing solution contained too much salt it would dry out and further irritate the eyes; if it contained too little, the eyes would retain too much of the water and become swollen. Washing the eyes flushes out substances that are causing the irritation and, as a result, the redness soon subsides. But if one continues to subject the eyes to situations that cause redness the eyes will quickly become bloodshot again.

Most eyedrops and eyewashes operate on this flushing principle. Another type of eyedrop (available only by prescription) adds epinephrine to the isotonic solution. This drug actually shrinks the swollen blood vessels while the isotonic solution is rinsing out the irritants. Epinephrine eyedrops are usually reserved for severe or longstanding cases of bloodshot eyes.

Tearing of the Eyes

Heavy tearing of the eyes is frequently due to the same irritants which caused bloodshot eyes. The eyes, realizing that there is an irritant present, try to wash it out by themselves by producing an increased amount of tears. Treatment consists of washing the eyes with the same simple isotonic solution used for bloodshot eyes. With the irritants removed, the eyes stop tearing.

When the irritation is caused by an allergy, eyewashes may not relieve the tearing. Identifying and controlling the underlying allergy with antihistamines, desensitizing shots, or in severe cases with cortisone will usually put a stop to the tearing. (See Chapter 7, "Skin Sensitivity.")

Constant, heavy tearing that does not respond to eyedrops or allergy treatments may be caused by a malfunction in the tear-producing apparatus. This is a serious medical problem and should be handled by an ophthalmologist (eye specialist).

The Eye Area

Puffy Lids and the Eyes

Allergies are a major cause of this eye problem. The allergic reaction causes fluid to leak out of the blood vessels. This fluid has a tendency to accumulate in the tissues of the eyelids, giving the eyes a swollen appearance. Identification of the allergy and its control will also control the eye swelling.

Acute infections of the eye area, such as sinusitis, cause an abrupt swelling of the eyes. Such conditions are frequently accompanied by fever, pain around the eyes and cheeks, and headache. These problems are treated with antibiotics, aspirin, and rest. When the infection subsides the swelling also disappears.

Many people notice that their eyes are swollen in the morning, but as the day progresses the swelling disappears. This can be caused by chronic sinus problems, allergic rhinitis, or a postnasal drip. All of these conditions may cause an accumulation of fluid in the eye area leading to swelling of the lids. During the day, when one is standing up and walking around, the fluid is able to drain out of the area. But when one is asleep, the fluid cannot drain and winds up in the lid area. Such problems are possibly the most frequent cause of puffy eyes and the simplest to control. A decongestant taken before going to sleep will reduce the amount of fluid produced. Raising the head of the bed six inches or more will help whatever fluid is produced to drain out of the sinuses and nose area so that it will not accumulate in the eyes.

Lines and Baggy Tissue Around the Eyes

The tone and flexibility of the skin around the eyes, like every other area of the skin, depend heavily on the health of the collagen fibers of the dermis. If the collagen has been stretched out of shape or loses its flexibility, the skin wrinkles and sags.

Collagen around the eyes is subjected to almost constant strain. Each time the eyes open and close, look up and down, widen in surprise, or squint at the sun, the collagen fibers are stretched. It is not surprising that the eye area is frequently the first to develop lines and wrinkles.

Damaged collagen is not the sole cause of the problem. Changes in the distribution of fat deposits around the eyes contribute to sagging and pouching of the skin in this area. The fat pads of the eye area are held in place by a membrane. As one grows older the membrane becomes weaker and the fat pads push through, bulging into the eyelids. They appear as loose baggy skin under the eyes and heavy overhanging upper lids.

Some cosmeticians suggest special exercises to strengthen the eye muscles to "resist" the pressure of the fat and thus avoid a bulge. While it is not clear whether (a) exercises do in fact strengthen the eye muscles and (b) whether strengthened muscles do hold back the fat pads (the fat pads lie on top of the muscle and it is difficult to see how the muscle could hold them back), the exercise movements to strengthen the eye muscles will place additional strain on the collagen, and further increase wrinkling in this particularly wrinkle-prone area. Baggy, lined eye areas are usually part of the aging process and their care and management are discussed thoroughly in Chapter 5, "Problems of the Mature Skin."

There are other instances where people in their twenties and thirties can have this type of problem. For instance, a too rapid weight loss can lead to slightly baggy skin. This bagging is particularly noticeable around the eyes.

People with puffy eyes caused by allergies are constantly stretching and straining the collagen fibers around the eyes. These people will develop loose, baggy skin around the eyes at an earlier age.

Reducing slowly and controlling chronic allergies and sinus problems are obviously the best ways to prevent the premature stretching of the skin. If the damage already exists, there is an operation that removes the excess skin of the lids and under the eyes, making the skin of the eyes look firm and smooth. This surgery is usually part of the overall face lift operation for aging skin. Most surgeons feel that if the eyes need help, so does the rest of the face (see pages 90–1). But in those cases where the skin around the eyes is prematurely aged by other factors, the eye operation alone is done.

Circles Under the Eyes

There are two major causes of dark circles under the eyes and it is possible for a person to have both of these underlying problems at once, which can make for very dark circles indeed.

First of all, note that the skin under the eyes is very thin. The blood supply running under this skin is visible, and these blood vessels give a bluish tone to the fine undereye tissue. Some people have especially thin skin, and this makes their blood vessels seem more prominent and the circles under their eyes even darker.

Many people notice that when they are tired the circles under their eyes look even darker. This is because the rest of the face is paler by contrast, and therefore the circles under their eyes stand out more.

In the same way, if you are anemic, your circles may appear more prominent. Correcting anemia or getting more sleep will make the rest of your face less pale and the circles under your eyes will be less prominent.

If your skin is on the pale side and you have prominent circles under your eyes, make sure that you:

1. Get plenty of rest.

2. Eat enough iron-rich food.

3. In order to decrease the contrast between pale skin and dark circles, use a circulation-stimulating face mask like those used for pale skin.

Dark circles can also be caused by melanin deposits in the delicate, thin-skinned areas beneath the eyes. In this case you want to discourage melanin production. The undereye area should be shielded from any contact with the sun. Wear a strong sunscreen cream or lotion around the eyes when going outdoors in daylight. Use sunglasses that cover the whole eye area.

It is very interesting to note that *stress* can cause an increase in melanin production. Severely ill patients often have deep rings under their eyes, which are thought to result from the situational stress of their physical and/or emotional state. It is possible that anxiety and overwork in an otherwise healthy person can cause the body to produce extra melanin.

Dark circles due to stress-induced melanin production are best handled by:

1. Avoiding direct sunlight on the eye areas, by the use of a sun cream that is a total sunscreen around the eyes, such as UVAL (Dome).

2. Wearing dark glasses that shield the entire eye area. Be sure that your sunglasses have truly polarized lenses, and not just decorative pale blue or pink glass lenses.

3. Getting plenty of rest and trying to relax.

As I mentioned earlier, it is possible that the circles under your eyes might be due, simultaneously, to both underlying causes —anemic pale skin and melanin-producing situations. In this case, you should combine all the corrective measures listed previously. Make certain that your anemia is corrected, use circulation-stimulating face masks, and take anti-sun precautions for the areas under your eyes.

Part Three / The Hair

11 / What the Hair Is Made of and How It Grows

What makes hair shiny?

Why is some hair dry?

What does a permanent wave do to your hair?

The answers to these and other questions lie in a basic understanding of the hair itself.

The Anatomy of a Hair Strand

Each strand of hair has three major layers (see Diagram 21, page 166). The outermost layer, the *cuticle*, is an overlapping series of cells arranged very much like shingles on a roof. The cuticle is made up of keratin, the same substance that forms the outermost layer of the skin. The cuticle prevents noxious chemicals from penetrating to the core of the hair and acts as a protective covering against excessive evaporation of water. Like skin, hair needs water to remain supple and shiny.

The second layer of the hair shaft, which lies immediately below the cuticle, is the *cortex*. The cortex contains the pigment granules that determine the color of the hair.

The innermost layer of the hair is called the *medulla*. Not very much is known about the biological function of this layer. Some scientists believe that the medulla acts as a carrier of food and oxygen to the other layers of the hair. However, the significance

Diagram 21.

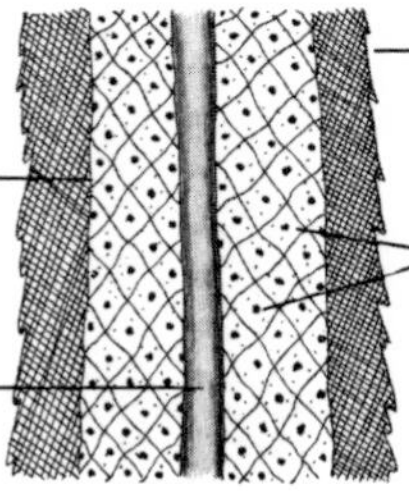

Cortex —

Cuticle

Melanin Granules

Medulla —

LONGITUDINAL SECTION OF HAIR SHAFT

and validity of this suggestion are still in doubt, and many perfectly normal and healthy hairs have fragmented or broken-up medullas, or no medulla at all. Contrary to what some experts say, a solid, intact medulla is not a sign of healthy hair, nor is the broken or fragmented medulla a sign of sick hair. Any product that claims to restore the medulla and thereby make the hair strong and healthy is a fraud.

How the Hair Grows

Each hair grows out of a single depression in the scalp called the follicle. A hair begins life as a clump of cells called the *papilla* at the bottom of the follicle. Beside supplying the basic cells for the hair, the papilla, with its many blood vessels, is a source of food and oxygen for the fully grown hair. The health and well-being of the hair is dependent on the circulation of the blood in the papilla. If the blood supply is decreased, the hair gets less food and oxygen and its appearance suffers. Decreased circulation can come about from the general slowdown of old age, from heart disease, or simply from improper scalp care. Proper brushing gives

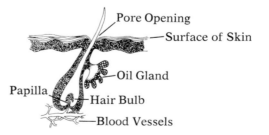

Pore Opening

Surface of Skin

Oil Gland

Papilla

Hair Bulb

Blood Vessels

Diagram 22. Hair Follicle in Scalp

a wonderful boost to the scalp's circulation, which increases the blood supply and makes the hair healthier and stronger.

When forming a hair, the cells of the papilla multiply and rearrange themselves to form the *hair bulb*. As the hair bulb increases in size, the cells change, stretching themselves to become the hair strand that can be seen projecting from the scalp. As these cells grow, they arrange themselves in the three separate layers described above—the tough outer coating of keratin called the cuticle, as well as the two inner layers, the medulla and the cortex.

The growth cycle of the human hair is a three-step process. In step one, the cells at the bottom of the follicle are busily growing and rearranging themselves into a new hair, which will eventually replace the older hair already in the follicle.

Diagram 23.

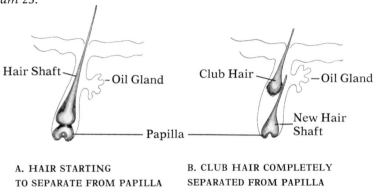

A. HAIR STARTING
TO SEPARATE FROM PAPILLA

B. CLUB HAIR COMPLETELY
SEPARATED FROM PAPILLA
The new hair is ready
to appear at the opening of the follicle.

This initial growth is a signal to the hair already in the follicle (which is the hair that is visible on the scalp) to loosen itself (step two) from the papilla and to move itself out of the follicle. This departing hair is called a *club hair*, and it is a dying hair.

In the third and final step the club hair falls out and the new hair moves up to take its place. This new hair continues to grow for two to six years. If it is pulled out early in this period, it can take quite a while before a new hair grows in to take its place, for no new hair is formed in the follicle beneath the scalp while a healthy shaft of hair is growing. However, if the club hair (old hair) comes out prematurely, the new hair already forming in the follicle will quickly replace the prematurely removed club hair.

The Oil Glands of the Scalp

The oil glands along the side of each hair follicle deposit *sebum* (oil) into the follicle. The sebum rises up the follicle and coats the hair with a thin layer of oil. This coating prevents excessive evaporation of water from the hair shaft, keeping it soft and flexible. The oil, in coating the hair, fills in the little cracks in the cuticle that make the hair look dull and dry. By filling in the cracks, the surface is made smooth and it reflects the light evenly. This causes the hair to look shiny.

The flow of oil from the glands in the scalp is influenced by the same factors that stimulate the oil glands in the skin. At the base of the control are the hormone secretions of two other glands —the androgens, secreted by the adrenal glands, and the estrogens, secreted by the ovaries. Usually these two hormones are in a fixed ratio; but if more of the androgens are produced, the balance is upset between these two hormones, which stimulates all of the body's oil glands, including those attached to the hair follicles, to secrete more oil. When this happens the hair suddenly seems to become oilier and limp.

Hair Characteristics

What Makes Hair Straight or Curly

Hair comes in three different shapes.

Straight hair usually has a round hair shaft (see Diagram 24A, page 169).

Wavy hair has an oval shape, resembling a baguette of French bread (see B).

Curly or kinky hair has a hair shaft that is flat when seen in cross-section (see C).

It appears that these differences in shape contribute to the different appearances of the hair.

The shape of the hair shaft, however, is not the whole story behind curly and straight hair. Recently it has been shown that each type grows differently in the follicle.

With straight hair the growth of the hair cells out of the

Diagram 24.

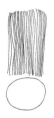
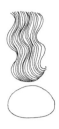
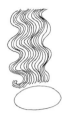

A. STRAIGHT HAIR
(cross-section below)

B. WAVY HAIR
(cross-section below)

C. KINKY OR CURLY HAIR
(cross-section below)

D. STRAIGHT-HAIR FOLLICLE   E. CURLY-HAIR FOLLICLE

papilla is equal all around the opening of the papilla. Thus the hair shaft grows evenly on both sides of the papilla (see Diagram 24D).

With curly hair the hair cells grow at *uneven rates* around the papilla. In this sort of growth, the hair shaft will begin to bend away from the side of the papilla where cell growth is most pronounced (see Diagram 24E). After a while, the side of the papilla that had been producing more cells slows down its growth rate, and the other side begins to grow more rapidly. The hair shaft now bends in the opposite direction. As soon as the hair has been bent a given amount to one side, it begins to bend to the other side, and so the cycle continues. This bending of the hair shaft continues throughout the life of the hair, causing waviness. The degree of curl is dependent on the length of the bending cycle. If the cycle is short, and there is a lot of bending, back and forth, the hair shaft will have many little waves. If the bending cycle is long, the waves are widely spaced, and the overall appearance is that of slightly wavy hair, with soft waves rather than full, tight curls.

There is no perfect hair type, as there may be with skin. Curly, straight, blond, black, long, and short hair have all been held by fashion at one time or another to be the most desirable kind of hair. However, shine, length, fullness, flexibility, and color contribute to the appearance of any type of hair, and the hair chemistry behind these attributes is worth knowing.

Shine

That quality of the hair called "shine" depends on the health of the cuticle, the outermost layer of the hair shaft. The cells of the cuticle are transparent and made up mostly of keratin. They form a flat, clear layer that reflects light on the surface of the hair shaft. This reflection is responsible for the hair's shine.

When the hair is healthy and shiny, these cells lie flat and tight along the shaft. When the hair has been damaged, these cells stand away from the rest of the hair shaft. The smooth, even surface is broken—light can no longer be reflected evenly from this surface, and the hair looks dull.

Many things can disrupt the cuticle of the hair. These include alkaline shampoos, which make the whole hair shaft swell. This swelling pushes out the cells of the cuticle, causing them to stand away from the hair shaft. If the alkaline substances are very harsh (like those used in permanent-waving and coloring), they can dissolve, some of the cuticle leaving pits and holes in the hair, which cause the hair to look dull.

Acidic substances, on the other hand, make the hair shaft tight and smooth. They shrink the hair shaft and encourage the cuticle cells to lie flat. These acidic substances also strengthen keratin. This is why acid-based products should be used on your hair.

The amount of oil on the hair also plays an important role in the shine of the hair. The natural oil secreted by the scalp coats

Diagram 25.

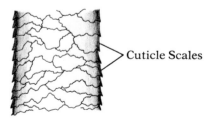

Cuticle Scales

SURFACE OF HAIR SHAFT

the strand of each hair with a smooth film of oil. This oil fills in cracks and creates an even, light-reflecting surface. While the oil coating is important, it cannot take the place of proper care of the hair. An oily hairdressing will give some shine to damaged hair but it will not restore flexibility, strength, and bounce.

Hair sprays and setting lotions dull the hair because they coat it with a sticky film. This film attracts dirt and dust easily, which settles on the hair. The presence of this dirt on the hair creates an irregular, bumpy surface on the shaft, causing poor light reflection and dull-looking hair.

Length

The length a hair can achieve varies from person to person. During the first two to four years of the average life span of an individual hair, the shaft can grow anywhere from twelve to thirty-six inches. Many people find that after the hair achieves a certain length, often shoulder length, the hair seems to stop growing. When hair reaches its absolute length, it lives for a while longer and then falls out. A new hair will grow only to this same length as well. The length a hair will grow can sometimes be increased with special care. Gentle brushing, mild shampoos, scalp massage, and avoiding bleach or cold waves will prevent hair from falling out before it has come of age, and thus increase its chances of achieving maximum growth.

Fullness

The relative thickness or thinness of one's head of hair depends on the diameter and shape of each individual hair as well as the total number of hairs on the head. Fine, thin hair obviously has the smallest diameter, while coarse hair has the thickest. Straight hair is usually smaller in diameter than curly hair.

The number of hairs on the head varies with the hair's color. On the average, blond hair has the narrowest hair shaft and needs the greatest number of hairs to give a respectable covering to the scalp. Red hair has the thickest hair shaft and requires fewer hairs to give the same impression of fullness as blond hair. The number of hairs necessary to give an average appearance of full-ness is:

$$Blond = 140,000 \text{ hairs/head}$$
$$Brown = 110,000 \text{ hairs/head}$$
$$Black = 108,000 \text{ hairs/head}$$
$$Red = 90,000 \text{ hairs/head}$$

Most people like the appearance a full head of hair gives and when people feel their hair is not thick enough, they will search for some way to increase the numbers of hairs on their head. This is futile, since the number of hairs is determined by the number of hair roots, which is fixed at birth. What can be done is to try to increase the width of the hairs already present and to preserve those that are growing. The hair strands can be increased in bulk with protein shampoos and conditioners, or by coloring, which swells the hair shaft.

Flexibility, Softness, and Bounce

These characteristics are all related to the water content of the hair and its effects on the health of the hair protein called keratin.

The flexibility and elasticity of the hair depend on how much water a hair contains. Healthy hair contains enough water to keep the keratin fiber firm and supple. This hair takes a set well and feels soft to the touch. If you pull on both ends, a healthy hair will stretch without breaking. However, if a hair loses water through too much processing or too much sun, the keratin fiber of the hair will no longer possess its natural elastic qualities. If you pull at this hair, it will not stretch, but will break off sharply; loss of water has caused it to become brittle. This hair feels brittle, refuses to take or hold a set, and has many split ends.

Color

The color of a hair depends on the amount and type of *melanin* (pigment) granules present in the cortex, the middle layer of the hair.

Red hair has a mixture of red and black pigments; blond

hair contains red and yellow pigments; sandy-brown hair contains red, brown, and black pigments; dark-brown hair contains simply more black pigment than does sandy-brown hair; finally, black hair contains even more black pigment than does dark-brown hair, and white hair has no pigment granules whatsoever.

Melanin is produced by the body through a fairly complex transformation of certain naturally occurring proteins under the action of specific enzymes found in the pigment-producing cells. The different colors of melanin pigments probably represent different stages of the development of melanin. First the yellow pigment is formed, then a specific enzyme produced by the body changes the yellow pigment to a red pigment. Another enzyme will then change the red pigment to a black pigment.

Not everyone has the ability to change the melanin to this whole spectrum of colors. Some people produce black pigment; they will have dark-brown or black hair depending on how much black pigment they produce. Other persons can only produce red and yellow pigments, and they will have blond or red hair. The ability to produce these pigments is determined by the enzymes present, and is an intimate part of a person's hereditary makeup. In the albino, the enzymes necessary for the formation of pigment are absent and therefore all pigments are absent.

The intensity and shade of the color of a woman's hair depends on the amounts of pigment found in the individual hairs. Flaming red hair has a great deal of red pigment, whereas pale-red hair has much less pigment.

Dull, faded color can be the result of an unsatisfactory mixture of melanin pigments. The combination of red, black, and golden pigments in certain proportions will result in a murky, dense brownish-blond color that looks drab and uninteresting, even when well cared for. There is nothing physically wrong with such hair other than the esthetic problem it creates.

The ability to produce different pigments is genetically determined. Nevertheless, more than any other features, hair color can be successfully changed with dyes and tints. Done properly and with care, this change will not damage the hair and can make a significant difference in your appearance.

12 / The Basics of Hair Care

Brushing and Combing

Proper brushing is absolutely essential for the hair and scalp. Brushing removes the loose scales accumulated on the scalp, and distributes the oil evenly throughout your hair. The oil provides a protection against excessive water evaporation, and fills in the tiny cracks in the hair shafts, making the hair smooth and shiny. In addition, combing and brushing stimulate blood circulation, which guarantees that each hair will get plenty of oxygen and food to insure its good health and long life. But the brushing ritual must be done correctly if it is to be of benefit.

The brush should be firm, with evenly spaced clumps of bristles. The bristles should be natural, animal bristles, not nylon. Natural bristles have rounded ends. Nylon bristles have squared off, sharp ends. These can cause cracks and splits in the hair. A particularly excellent brush has the bristles set in a layer of rubber that is in turn attached to the body of the brush.

A comb should be firm enough not to bend easily with pressure. The teeth should be evenly spaced. They should not be extremely close together; too fine a comb puts too much strain on the hair.

Both the comb and the brush should be washed frequently. A good rule of thumb is that every other time you wash your hair, wash the comb and the brush. Fill the sink with lukewarm water. Add a tablespoonful of liquid shampoo and two to three drops of ammonia and swish the comb and brush through the soapy water.

Let them sit in the water for ten minutes. Drain the water from the sink and rinse both the brush and the comb in plenty of lukewarm water. Dry the brush off with a towel.

Smashing the brush down over the hair will damage the scalp and injure the individual hairs, breaking them off and splitting the ends. Brushing should be done with a firm and regular stroke. Concentrate mainly on the scalp. Pull your brush through the hair close to the scalp in a smooth, even stroke. Repeat this until the scalp feels warm and tingly.

Then, holding the hair firmly with your free hand at about ear length, run your brush through the loose hair. If your hair is very long (more than six inches below shoulder length) do not pull the brush through to the ends of the hair. Instead, run the brush down about the first eight inches of hair from the scalp. Then, holding the hair at this spot with your free hand, run the brush down another eight inches toward its ends, continuing this staggered-section brushing until all the hair is brushed. This use of the free hand as a holding anchor during brushing produces a minimum of strain on the hair roots, and prevents too many hairs from being needlessly pulled out.

When the hair on your scalp and the very long strands of hair have been brushed, put your head down and brush the hair from the nape of your neck toward the top of the head. Brush in short, regular, firm strokes all around the back of the head.

This type of heavy brushing should be done before you wash your hair, once or twice weekly. If you wash more frequently, still brush this thoroughly only twice a week. If done every day, heavy brushing will make hair too oily and take out too much of the set. After washing and a set, gently brush out and smooth the hair into place. Once a day pass a brush through your hair in a firm, smooth manner. Do not try to make the scalp tingle, or to reach all parts of the hair. Just brush the top of the head and surface hair to distribute oil and remove dust and dirt. Ten or twelve strokes should do it.

The combing of hair should be done with the same care. Do not pull and yank at a tangle. It will tear out too much hair. If a tangle is really that troublesome, spray it with a dilute solution of cream rinse and comb it through. The cream rinse contains a substance (see page 179) that softens the hair and releases the tangle.

· · ·

Shampooing

A good washing of the hair removes old dull oil, loose scalp flakes, and sooty dirt, and it relaxes the hair, which makes it easier to set. Every shampoo should consist of a thorough brushing, two sudsings of soap, a conditioner, followed by setting or careful blow-drying to give style and shape to the hair. The type of shampoo and conditioner to be used depends on the particular kind of hair, but the basic aims and techniques of a shampoo are the same for all kinds of hair.

There are really only two kinds of shampoos: those made of soap and those made with detergents. Most commercially available shampoos today are detergents.

Soap Shampoos

Soap shampoos have a tendency to be very alkaline, a factor that can break down the hair protein. When used with hard water (which is what most of the water throughout the world is), soap shampoos leave a deposit of soap and mineral scum in the hair. This can make the hair look very dull. It is also hard to modify the qualities of a soap shampoo to make it less drying or better cleaning.

Detergent Shampoos

Detergent shampoos, while they might sound harsh and unnatural, are really a better product. They are usually less alkaline than soap shampoos. They do not leave a dulling film on the hair, and they take readily to the addition of new chemicals to give the shampoo better properties, such as more cleaning power and less static after washing.

The designation of a shampoo for dry, normal, or oily hair depends simply on the shampoo's degreasing abilities. Those formulated for oily hair contain larger amounts of grease-dissolving solvents than the shampoos made for dry hair.

Both soap and detergent shampoos come in three forms: liquid, liquid cream, or paste. You should choose whichever is best suited to your hair.

Liquid and Liquid-cream Shampoos

Liquid shampoos are usually clear and transparent, and are gold or greenish in color. They rarely contain any "additional" oils. This is a good shampoo for normal or oily hair. Colored, waved, or dry hair needs a milder shampoo. Liquid-cream shampoos are white, thick liquids. They are usually detergents with soap added to thicken and whiten them. They frequently contain additional oils such as lanolin. They are too rich for oily hair but are good for dry or processed hair.

Paste Shampoos

Paste shampoos are thick white creams that come in a jar. They also contain additional oils and are more concentrated than liquid-cream shampoos. They can be used successfully by people with normal hair, but are too rich for people with oily hair and too alkaline for dry hair.

Shampoos with Additives

There are almost an infinite number of additives that are put into a shampoo. Among the more common ones are: protein, herbal additives, balsam, lemon, and egg.

PROTEIN: This protein is usually derived from the cartilage and joints of cows or pigs. The hair picks up a coating of protein from the shampoo. This coating strengthens the hair and fills in cracks in the cuticle caused by strong alkaline chemicals such as those used in dyeing, waving, or straightening. The layer of protein also makes the hair look thicker. Protein shampoos are excellent for thin, limp, or damaged hair. They are not necessary for normal hair; they do not help dry hair; and can make oily hair limp soon after shampooing.

HERBAL ADDITIVES: Some herbal shampoos are based on a single herb while others contain a whole garden of different plants.

Herbs are one of the few natural substances that can maintain some of their potency during the manufacturing process. However, it is vital to know the value of the herbs you are using. Some, like camomile, can brighten the hair and make it shiny. Others, like comfrey root, can soothe an itchy, inflamed scalp. Still others, like parsley and lemon balm, do absolutely nothing. Before buying an herbal shampoo check the Glossary at the back of this book for the value of the herbs that it contains, to make sure it is the best shampoo for your hair type.

BALSAM: Balsam is a thick, sticky substance extracted from the bark of tropical trees. Like protein, it forms a coating on the hair strand, giving strength and thickness to the hair.

LEMON: Shampoos containing lemon juice or citric acid, which is the active ingredient in lemon juice, are especially good for oily hair. They have the ability to remove excess oil from the hair and scalp without making the hair stiff and dull. They will, however, make dry and processed hair bushy and drier.

EGG: The egg in an egg shampoo has no effect on the appearance of the hair. The hair cannot utilize the protein in the egg and therefore any value of such a shampoo lies in its other ingredients, such as the soap, the emulsifiers, and the oils. The higher price of egg shampoo is not justified, since it does not especially help any type of hair.

ACID pH OR BALANCED pH: While pH is not actually an additive in itself, it is the end result of additives. A balanced pH such as is achieved in certain shampoos has value for dry and processed hair.

Most shampoos are somewhat alkaline, and alkaline substances have a tendency to make the hair shaft swollen and flaky. This can make even normal hair look dull and feel stiff, and can cause processed (bleached or permanent) hair to become extremely dry, brittle, and lifeless. Acid or balanced pH shampoos can shrink the cuticle and make the hair shaft stronger and shinier. These shampoos are good for normal hair and are an absolute necessity for dry and processed hair. While they improve the health and strength of every type of hair, they do not have enough grease-cutting action for oily hair, and leave it dull and limp.

Conditioning

The proper conditioner will correct many hair problems. There are five different types of conditioners and each type does a different job. You should pick the one that answers your hair needs.

Cream Rinses

These are thick, creamy solutions usually diluted with water before use, and they are frequently advertised as detanglers. Their active ingredients are quaternary ammonium salts; these chemicals can break some of the hair's own chemical bonds and soften the hair. These rinses are excellent for naturally dry and bushy hair, but make normal or oily hair limp—although they may be advertised for oily hair. Because of their alkalinity, they can hurt damaged, dyed, or colored hair.

Herbal Rinses

The value of herbal rinses depends on what kind of chemicals are used as a base, and what herbs this rinse contains. While many herbs do retain their potency in a cosmetic, the properties of a base can overpower the activity of the herbs. For example, while camomile makes dull oily hair shinier, if it is put into a thick cream rinse, the hair will become dull and limp. Cosmetics based on herb formulas may contain many different types of herbs, some of which are effective, some of which are useless, and finally some of which may cause allergic reactions. For these reasons, this book does not recommend any commercial conditioner based on herbs. While some might be effective, it is often impossible to figure out which one would be best for your type of hair. It is best to stick with a product whose value can be accurately determined from a knowledge of the ingredients.

Nevertheless, fresh infusions of certain herbs can be excellent for some hair problems. Clover blossom, cornflower, camomile, and orange pekoe tea can brighten and soften oily hair. Fennel (which is slightly antiseptic) and nettle (which contains vitamin A) are good for dandruff. All herbal infusions are made and used in the same way.

TO PREPARE HERBAL INFUSIONS

1. Steep one tablespoonful of the herbs you have selected in eight ounces of boiling water for thirty minutes, strain, and *cool*.

2. Pour into hair and work into scalp.

3. Let remain for fifteen to twenty minutes.

4. Rinse out with lukewarm water.

Protein Conditioners

These conditioners act in much the same way as protein shampoos. The protein forms a coating on the outside of the hair shaft, filling in cracks in the cuticle and making a watertight shield that helps hair retain moisture. Protein conditioners are excellent for thin hair, since they add bulk by making each hair strand a little thicker with its coating. They are also excellent for strengthening damaged or processed hair. Dry, normal, or oily hair does not get any value from them. Protein conditioners are available in cream form, thin fluids, and lotions.

Body Builders

These are thin, clear fluids frequently packaged as individual treatments. They are made up of water and shellac and are basically a dilute solution of hair spray. They give considerable body to the hair . . . but at a price. They make the hair sticky and dull. They can cause dry hair to look drier and bushier, and they can make oily hair oilier and lank soon after washing. With all these drawbacks they are still the best conditioners for thin, limp hair.

Cream Conditioners

These are thick creams that are applied to the hair, left on for several minutes, then washed out. They are designed for dry, processed, or damaged hair and do a good job of restoring the water balance of the hair. They are not quite as good as protein conditioners, but usually are much cheaper. They will only make normal or oily hair flat, limp, and dull.

A BASIC PROCEDURE FOR SHAMPOOING
AND CONDITIONING THE HAIR

1. Brush your hair thoroughly as described on pages 174–5. Follow this up with a scalp massage (pages 185–6).

2. Wet your hair completely with warm water. Do not let the water strike your head forcefully. It can strain and tangle the hair if it hits the scalp with too great a pressure.

3. Apply the shampoo, a bit at a time, all over your head. Starting at the top of the head rub in some shampoo; then apply some around the ears, the back of the head, and the front of the hair line, rubbing it as you apply it.

4. When all parts of your head are covered with shampoo, start massaging the head, working the shampoo into the scalp with the balls of your fingers, not your fingernails.

5. Work the shampoo into the long part of your hair, but don't try to wash the ends too energetically; it will only make them dry and brittle.

6. Rinse out your hair and repeat the sudsing once again. Remember, do not use a strong blast of water to rinse out your hair; it will hurt the hair. Rinse.

7. Pour your conditioner on now.

8. Rinse out the conditioner with warm water.

9. Wrap your head in a soft towel. Press towel gently against your head. Do not rub your hair to dry it, since at this point your hair is at its most fragile. Rubbing puts great strain on the hair and can break it off, causing unnecessary hair loss.

10. Comb your hair through *gently*.

11. The hair is now ready for setting.

. . .

Setting the Hair

All parts of the hair are made of protein. The protein molecules are arranged in organized patterns and are held in those patterns by two kinds of chemical bonds—hydrogen bonds (H-bonds) and sulfur bonds (S-bonds). The formations these molecules and their chemical bonds take determine the wave of the hair. As mentioned earlier, it is believed that the waviness of the hair is determined by the manner in which the hair grows out of the follicle. This shape seems to be maintained by these chemical bonds.

In straight hair, all the bonds are at right angles to the hair shaft as you can see in A, Diagram 26. With wavy hair, on the other hand, the bonds are found at different angles along the shaft of the hair. *Setting* and *permanent-waving* consists of breaking these bonds, arranging them into a new shape, and reforming new bonds to "freeze" this shape.

Hydrogen bonds are the ones that are broken and re-formed bonds are very *strong* ones. Water, heat, mild alkaline solutions, even the pressure of combing your hair will break the weak hydrogen bonds. Sulfur bonds, on the other hand, require boiling water or very strong alkaline solutions before they are broken.

Hydrogen bonds are the ones that are broken and re-formed when you *wash and set* your hair. Sulfur bonds are broken and re-formed during *permanent-waving* and *straightening*.

When setting your hair, you want the wave to last three or four days, your hair to be soft and shiny, and to avoid any damage to the hair. To achieve these goals, follow these

Diagram 26.

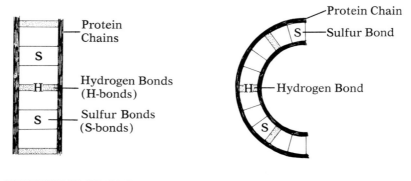

A. STRUCTURE OF STRAIGHT HAIR   B. STRUCTURE OF CURLY HAIR

RULES FOR SETTING THE HAIR

1. Always start by breaking the hydrogen bonds. You can accomplish this by wetting the hair thoroughly with warm water; by steaming the hair over your sauna; or by applying hot rollers. Newly washed hair always takes a wave best, because its hydrogen bonds have been freshly broken during washing.

2. Use a setting lotion if the program for your type of hair calls for it. (Each type of hair will be discussed separately, in Chapter 13.) Unprocessed hair (that is, hair that has not been recently dyed, colored, waved, or straightened) can benefit from a slightly alkaline preparation. Such preparations will make the hair more porous and therefore admit more water into the hair shafts, thus breaking more H-bonds. The more bonds are broken and then re-formed, the better and longer-lasting the set will be. Processed hair is porous enough for this to happen naturally. It absorbs plenty of water, and is too fragile to be treated with anything alkaline. Use an acid-based setting lotion for processed hair. All setting lotions, acid or alkaline, contain some kind of gum or resin. This coats the hair with a water-resistant shield. By protecting the hair from outside moisture, it keeps the set in longer. Even the moisture in the air is enough to act on the H-bonds, and break them, relaxing the set.

3. Stretch each strand of hair before putting it on rollers. This will relax the protein chain in the hair, making it easier for the hair to re-form itself into a new shape. Without this stretching, the set will be much weaker and looser, because the hairs did not have a chance to restructure themselves. However, do not stretch your hair so tight that the roots and scalp hurt. That can cause weakening, breaking, and loss of hair.

4. Be sure your hair is completely dry when it is removed from the rollers. Without total drying, new bonds are not completely formed and the set will soon collapse.

5. When setting your hair, divide your scalp into two sections so that both sides of your head are equal. This way the newly formed H-bonds are symmetrical over both sides of

your scalp, resulting in a hair style that is smooth and even.

6. Do not sleep on rollers. The pressure of the rollers against the scalp will interfere with circulation. It will put the hair under too much of a strain to be stretched and rolled for eight hours; finally, it will result in uneven pressures being exerted on the hair and cause an uneven set.

7. Fast drying with a hot-air dryer is the best method. Always be sure, though, to put the dryer on *cool* for the last five minutes of drying time to evaporate any perspiration formed on the scalp due to the hot dryer. This perspiration is enough moisture to break the hydrogen bonds and weaken the set.

8. Brush the set well. This will add shine and softness to the hair. It will relax the waves into natural-looking curves.

A BASIC PROCEDURE
FOR SETTING THE HAIR

1. Brush your hair well.
2. Shampoo thoroughly and condition.
3. Pat your hair gently with a towel. *Do not rub*.
4. Spray on a setting lotion.
5. Comb your hair through.
6. Section your hair and hold it with clips.
7. Take about an inch of hair, stretch it, and roll it on rollers. Use end papers if troubled by split ends.
8. Dry your hair thoroughly under the dryer.
9. For the last five minutes of this drying, turn the dryer down to *cool*.
10. Take the rollers out carefully. Unwind each one separately. Do not tear rollers out of your hair. Pulling too hard can inadvertently pull out clumps of hair.
11. Brush out your hair and arrange it in the desired style.

Electric Rollers

If time is short, electric rollers can give a good, if somewhat short-lived, set. The heat in the rollers breaks the bonds in the hair.

Then, as the roller cools, the hair re-forms its bonds while wrapped around the roller. The set does not last as long as a regular set. A thorough shampoo and set breaks far more bonds and lets them re-form more thoroughly than do the electric rollers.

The hot-mist roller will do an even better job of breaking the bonds and will give a longer-lasting set. Furthermore, the water in the mist prevents the hair from losing too much moisture, as will sometimes happen with the ordinary hot roller. This is not vital to the health of normal or oily hair but can make quite a bit of difference in the appearance of dry or processed hair.

Massaging

Scalp massage is an essential part of any hair care routine. Thoroughly and properly performed, massage stimulates the scalp's circulation, helps to remove loose dandruff flakes, and ensures the hair's continued good health.

The hair root is fed by a network of tiny blood capillaries. These blood vessels bring oxygen and food to the hair root and carry away carbon dioxide (CO_2) and other metabolic waste products. If the circulation is poor and the blood cannot readily travel through the vessels, the hair root suffers. The root no longer receives enough nutrients and the waste products accumulate in the tissues. Under these circumstances the cells of the hair root grow very slowly and may even die. When this happens, new hairs are no longer formed, and the existing hairs die. This can lead to a noticeable thinning of the hair, which may or may not be permanent.

As one grows older, the circulation of the whole body slows down. This will affect the scalp's circulation and can be a factor in the decline of the hair's appearance after the age of fifty.

Individuals with oily hair are particularly prone to a sluggish scalp circulation. The oil and dead cells of the scalp combine to form a solid film of debris on the scalp surface. This layer hardens and sticks to the scalp. In effect, it "strangles" the scalp's circulation. This condition is called *tight scalp*. Just about the only way to alleviate this problem is with scalp massage.

Proper scalp stimulation is rarely achieved, even by people who take good care of their hair. It takes ten to fifteen minutes of thorough brushing to get the scalp to feel warm and tingly—a sign that the circulation has been stimulated. A good scalp massage will accomplish the same thing in two to three minutes.

The best way to massage the scalp is with an electric scalp vibrator. Some of these vibrators are equipped with a heating unit. The warmth increases the vibrator's effect on the circulation and can also encourage oil-gland secretion. These vibrators are particularly useful for people with dry or damaged hair.

Electric Scalp Vibrators

These range in price from about eight to thirty dollars. Oster makes a plain vibrator for about eight dollars and a heated vibrator for about fourteen dollars. It is not necessary to spend a great deal of money for this device. A reliable inexpensive machine is adequate.

A scalp massage should be performed at least twice weekly. It does not replace the brushing done before a shampoo, since this brushing picks up the loose scales on the scalp and removes them. Massage only increases the circulation; it does not remove loose scales.

A BASIC PROCEDURE
FOR MASSAGING THE SCALP

1. Start the massage at the scalp line. Rub the vibrator on the front of the head and around the ears until this area of the scalp tingles.

2. Now rub the vibrator over the top of the head until tingly.

3. Bend your head forward and rub the vibrator over the back of the head and the neck, as well as behind the ears. Your scalp should feel warm and glowing all over.

13 / Major Hair Problems

Oily Hair

Oily hair is caused by the same conditions that cause oily skin. The hair, of course, is not producing the oil. It is coming from the scalp, which is rich in oil-producing glands.

The oil production of these glands is controlled by the ratio of two types of hormones that circulate in the blood, the estrogens and the androgens. Usually, a fixed ratio of these hormones is produced by the adrenal glands and the ovaries.

During puberty, however, this hormone balance changes radically, which is necessary for the normal maturation occurring at that time. In women, this process includes the forming of the breasts, the beginning of menses, and a host of transformations involving the bones and body metabolism in general. When these changes in hormones occur, the new balance stimulates the oil glands to produce much more oil, and both the skin of the face and the scalp become noticeably oilier.

After puberty the hormone balance usually stabilizes and the skin becomes far less oily. But the hair can remain prone to oiliness for many more years. While the exact cause of this long-lived oil activity is not known, there are many successful treatments that can control this problem.

When freshly washed and set, oily hair has a lovely sheen. However, left to its own devices it loses its set fairly quickly, and within two days becomes stringy, greasy, and limp. It must be washed very frequently, in some cases every other day, to avoid a lank oily look. Oily hair is especially prone to dandruff.

A PROFILE OF OILY HAIR

1. Do you have to wash your hair at least twice a week?
2. Does your set fall rather quickly?
3. Does damp, hot weather make your hair especially lank?
4. Do you have dandruff?
5. Do you have, or you have had, acne problems?
6. Is your skin now oily, or was it oily during your twenties and thirties?

In Chapter 4, a distinction was made between teenage acne, adult acne, and plain oily skin. Hair is much simpler. Oily hair is simply oily, and the approach to its care does not depend on your age. The oilier the hair is, the more frequently you can treat it, but basically it is the same method.

The Care of Oily Hair

Contrary to popular belief, oily hair should be thoroughly brushed to promote its valuable sheen, and the scalp should be massaged to promote circulation. The scalp still needs a good supply of blood to maintain the growth of hair. If the hair's circulation is impaired, the hair will not grow well and will fall out. What you have to do is minimize the oiliness, but not at the expense of the sheen of your hair or the health of your scalp.

Oily hair needs a shampoo especially formulated for oily hair. This does not mean that the shampoo contains less oil, but simply that its soap is strong and removes oil from the hair. Lemon shampoos are frequently good for oily hair, since lemon has good degreasing properties.

Balsam and protein shampoos do not help the appearance of oily hair, since they both leave a coating on the hair that makes the oily hair limp and sticky.

There are very few commercial conditioners that are helpful for oily hair. They all contain too many substances like oil, glycerin, or wax that will make the hair limp, dull, and oily very soon after shampooing. The best conditioner for oily hair is one you can make yourself out of fresh lemon juice. (Reconstituted lemon juice is good in a pinch, but fresh lemon juice actually works better.) Simply add the strained juice of one lemon to a cup of lukewarm water. After shampooing, pour on the lemon juice rinse, work it into the scalp and hair, then rinse it out with cool water. The lemon juice has a wonderful effect on oily hair. It has an astringent action that will temporarily close the scalp's pores, not allowing as much oil to seep out of the pores; in addition, it will dissolve any soap or grease left in the hair, leaving a brilliant shine to each strand. Furthermore, because of the acidity the cuticle will be tightened and smooth, making the hair soft and manageable.

Setting lotions make a set last longer, but since they contain oil and resins, they can make the hair sticky and oily and should not be used.

A PROGRAM OF CARE FOR OILY HAIR

Shampoo (twice weekly): Dissolve three tablespoonfuls of epsom salts in almost one half cup of liquid shampoo (the epsom salts act as a magnet, soaking up the oil from the hair). When the humidity is high, reduce the amount of epsom salts to one tablespoonful for about a half cup of shampoo.

1. Apply one tablespoonful of this mixture to dry hair.

2. Massage in well.

3. Rinse with cool water.

4. Shampoo again, this time with plain shampoo (no epsom salts).

5. Rinse out well. Blot excess water from hair.

6. Apply a lemon rinse and work it into the scalp and hair; let it remain for ten minutes. Now rinse out gently. Blot dry, comb, and set.

7. Try not to use hair spray on oily hair. It just makes it stickier and prone to collect dirt and grease.

. . .

Special Problems of Oily Hair

DANDRUFF: Oily hair is especially prone to dandruff. Oil on the scalp makes the cells of the scalp stick together and fall off in large clumps. These clumps are what we know as dandruff flakes.

Fortunately, oily hair is also strong hair, and you can use the strongest sulfur dandruff shampoos available. Many strong sulfur shampoos are available only by a doctor's prescription. Certain of them, such as SEBULEX by Westwood, can be purchased without a prescription. Check the label of any dandruff shampoo; sulfur is considered a biologically active ingredient, and must by law be listed on the package label.

See the section on pages 198–201 for a detailed program of dandruff control.

THE SUN AND OILY HAIR: Excess sun exposure is as bad for the hair as it is for the skin, but with oily hair, too much sun will not cause nearly as much damage as it does to dry or processed hair. Therefore, women with oily hair need not take the precaution of wearing a hat or a scarf each time they go out in the sun.

The sun will, however, stimulate the oil glands to produce more oil than is normal. Because of this, it will be necessary to wash the hair more often when there is frequent exposure to the sun.

Dry Hair

Dry hair can develop in four different ways. There is naturally dry hair; dryness due to processing (such as tinting, waving, straightening); coarse frizzy hair; and the dryness of graying hair.

Naturally Dry Hair

Naturally dry hair is due basically to lack of water. In this condition the oil glands of the scalp do not produce enough oil to coat the hair and prevent the evaporation of water from each strand. Without water, the hairs have a tendency to become stiff, "flyaway," and dull. There is no evidence that lack of oil in naturally dry youthful hair and skin is due to hormonal problems; it is probably the result of other factors that influence oil production. For example, there may be a smaller than average number of oil glands on the scalp, or the glands may be present in adequate numbers but individually may be producing small quantities of oil.

Naturally dry hair is fairly rare in young women. If it should occur in a young person it is usually accompanied by naturally dry facial skin. Untreated dry hair in a young person is frequently slightly curly or wavy, and often occurs in the darker shades of hair.

This kind of hair in this age group holds a set well and for a long time. It does not easily get stringy or oily and needs to be shampooed only once weekly or even every ten days to be well groomed. It is usually fairly thick, healthy hair, and normal care will keep it looking very good. However, because it is already dry, it has a greater tendency to lose water from processing than does normal or oily hair. Therefore, greater care must be taken during and after processing to prevent hair damage that might result from excessive water loss.

Dry hair of this type can be accompanied by "dry scalp dandruff." The dry scalp produces very little oil. Without a layer of oil, there is no shield against excessive evaporation of water, and the top layer of cells on the scalp loses a great deal of moisture. When this happens the cells flake away, no longer able to anchor themselves to the scalp. They fall off in clumps that we know as dandruff. This dandruff is quite different from that seen with oily hair, where the dandruff is formed by clumps of excess cells pasted together by oil.

The best way to treat this type of dry hair is to provide a protective coating or shield on the hair and scalp to compensate for the absence of a natural oil coating. Watertight shields for dry hair include the plant resin substances such as balsam, which coats the hair with a plastic-like layer that fills in tiny cracks and seals in water, and silicone, which forms a water-repelling barrier on the outside surface of the hair shaft, not allowing the water to escape.

Naturally dry hair, while it lacks water, is not weak like dry processed hair. Therefore you can use a cream rinse that contains quaternary ammonium salts; this will soften the dry hair strand and make it smoother and more manageable. A good cream rinse for dry hair should contain a shielding ingredient, such as balsam or silicone, some oil, and the quaternary ammonium salts. Two such products are ALMAY CREME RINSE and BRECK CREME RINSE.

The shampoo for dry hair should be gentle and contain lanolin, or a vegetable oil such as olive oil. Cream or paste shampoos are better than liquid shampoos because they contain more oil. An example of this type is LUSTRE CREME by Colgate-Palmolive. Protein shampoos are not necessary. They are usually more expensive than plain shampoos and the extra cost will not give better results. Save the protein hair products for the times you really need them.

Naturally dry hair does not need a setting lotion to maintain a good set. These products contain a resin or plastic-like substance that coats the hair, shielding the hair from outside humidity. Dry hair has little enough water, and a watertight shield will just make it dry and bushy and unmanageable.

A PROGRAM OF CARE FOR NATURALLY DRY HAIR

WEEKLY SHAMPOO

1. Wet hair and rub in shampoo.
2. Give head two thorough rinsings.
3. Rinse out well and blot off excess moisture.
4. Apply regular strength cream rinse according to directions.
5. Rinse out; blot off excess moisture.
6. Set hair while wet. Dry under medium heat.
7. Brush out to relax set.

Dry Hair After Processing

Processing (coloring, waving, straightening) and sunburn can cause normal hair to become extremely dry. The chemicals used in processing are extremely alkaline and they leach out water from the hair, making it brittle and dull. The sun will also dehydrate the hair with the same result.

At the same time this hair is losing water, its protein structure is changing, breaking apart. Naturally dry hair, while it lacks water, is still strong healthy hair. Processed hair, because it has lost some of its protein structure and water content, is *weak* hair. It becomes extremely brittle and rigid, the ends split and fray, it refuses to take a set, and it looks dull. Hair in this state must have both its water restored and its protein strength increased.

It is impossible to reconstruct a protein as complicated as hair, as some cosmetic companies would have us believe their products do. Rebuilding protein and increasing the growth rate of cells are (right now) something out of science fiction. But protein shampoos and conditioners do deposit a layer of protein *on* the hair, which fills in the cracks in the cuticle (the outermost layer of the hair), making the surface of the hair smooth and intact.

These added proteins provide support for the existing hair protein structures, much in the same way that a scaffolding supports a sagging wall. Many substances have the ability to coat the hair and provide some support, but the hair has the greatest affinity for proteins and retains them the best of all the reconditioning substances.

All types of hair can sustain dryness and damage from processing, even oily hair. It is not unusual to see a young girl with oily hair that has been damaged from too many color treatments. The hair nearest the scalp is quite oily, while the rest of the hair is dry and brittle. In these circumstances the whole head of hair should be treated as though it were dry and damaged; however, the weekly shampoo treatment should be increased to twice weekly to take care of the excess oil.

The fact that oily hair can show processing damage demonstrates that dry hair suffers from more than just a lack of oil. The harsh chemicals of processing remove the protective oil coating and also weaken the hair protein. Replacing this layer of oil with an oily dressing does not repair the protein damage or feed the hair water it has lost. An oily hairdressing can be a nice addition when the set is finished, but it should never be a substitute for proper shampooing and conditioning.

Processed hair is very fragile and cannot be treated like any other types of dry hair. It is as prone to dandruff as any other hair condition. The scalp is often quite dry and flakes off readily. Because the hair seems so brittle and stiff, many women are reluctant to wash it for fear of increasing dryness. This lack of washing leads to a buildup of dead cells, which in turn leads to the shedding of clumps of cells in the form of dandruff scales.

Processed hair is too weak to undergo treatment with sulfur-containing anti-dandruff shampoos. Sulfur attacks the keratin protein of the hair, which causes destruction of the hair itself and increases the chance of breakage. In cases of severely damaged hair due to processing, a sulfur shampoo can cause a section of the hair to dissolve into an amorphous insoluble gel, forming a tangled blob that has to be cut out of the rest of the hair.

Cream rinses are also too strong for processed hair. They contain hair-softening chemicals that can weaken already fragile hair and lead to hair breakage. Protein and acid rinses do a much better job of returning flexibility and bounce to this type of dry hair.

Acid shampoos give the very best results. Products with an acid pH are a must for damaged, dry hair. The strongly alkaline chemicals of the processing have left the hair swollen and the protein weakened. The acidity of reconditioning products will shrink the hair shaft back to normal size and firm up the protein.

Detailed programs for the care of processed hair will be found in Chapter 15.

Curly, Coarse, "Dry" Hair

Extremely curly, coarse hair can masquerade as dry hair. This kind of hair feels rough, stands stiffly away from the head, has little shine, and is almost impossible to style. It can appear with any color of hair and any skin type. Coarse, curly hair is *not* dry hair, and to treat it as such will not lead to any improvement in its appearance.

Coarse, curly hair has a very strong, thick hair shaft. It is extremely healthy hair. The hairs themselves have flexibility and elasticity, two vital signs of well-conditioned hair. But the hair is so firm and so solidly fixed in its curly formation that it stands away from the head, like a stiff brush.

The molecular bonds that hold the protein molecules in their curved positions are much more resistant to change than the same bonds in any other type of hair. The average shampoo and set that re-forms the bonds of other types of hair has little effect on coarse, curly hair.

Coarse, curly hair must be softened and the molecular bonds relaxed in order for it to be shiny and manageable. The most permanent way of doing this is by chemical hair straightening. Thioglycolic acid, the same substance used in cold-waving, is also used to straighten the hair. It softens the hair shaft and relaxes the molecular bonds so that the hair will now fall straight and flat on the head.

It is interesting to note that people who have their hair straightened notice that it subsequently seems quite oily and has to be washed often. The chemical processing has not made their hair oily; their scalp has always produced a great deal of oil, but the hair was so stiff and wiry that the oil did not seem to affect the hair as much. (For a more complete discussion on straightening, see Chapter 15, pages 252–7.)

Chemical hair straightening causes many of the same problems associated with cold-waving. It is a nuisance to do, it has to be repeated frequently, it is expensive, and, finally, it can lead to hair damage. Many people who have coarse, curly hair do not want completely straight hair; all they want is more attractive curly hair. For these people, and for those who do not want the bother of hair straightening, there is a simple and easy program that can be followed at home and can provide nice results.

Here is the problem to be solved: The hard and coarse hair must be softened. The bonds are very firm and tough and must be relaxed. In most of the other areas of hair care, the use of acid pH shampoos and conditioners was strongly recommended. In those situations, the hair shafts were made firmer and the bonds strengthened. This is precisely what should not be done for curly, coarse hair. For this type of hair, alkaline-based hair products must be used. These will soften the hair, make it silkier, and encourage the strong molecular bonds to relax, thus making the hair less curly.

A PROGRAM OF CARE FOR CURLY, COARSE, "DRY" HAIR

The shampoo should be plain, designed for normal hair, and contain absolutely no additives—such as herbs, balsam, or special oils.

Curly, coarse hair is made for cream rinse. The rinse contains hair-softening ingredients that will help relax the hair. Use a simple product—again, no fancy additives. Examples of this type are TAME by Toni and BRECK CREME RINSE.

1. Wet your head with very warm water, as the heat will relax the tight molecular bonds of the hair.

2. Add shampoo, work in well, rinse with very warm water.

3. Repeat the sudsing.

4. Make up a *triple-strength* cream rinse using hot water. If the manufacturer says to use one capful of the rinse to a cup of water, use three capfuls to one cup of water.

5. Pour this mixture over your head. You might wrap your head in SARAN WRAP to conserve heat and moisture, which will help the cream rinse do its job. In any event, leave the rinse on for fifteen minutes.

6. Rinse the hair out well with more warm water, as hot as you can stand.

7. Blot off excess moisture.

8. Set your hair on rollers. *Always* set this type of hair. At this point, your hair is quite relaxed and amenable to taking on a new shape. If you don't set it, it will bounce back to its old wild ways and the whole treatment will have been wasted.

9. Dry your hair under a hot dryer.

10. After removing the rollers from the hair, rub a dab of hairdressing like VITAPOINTE (Clairol) or ALBERTO VO5 cream hairdressing between the palms of your hands and then run your hands through the hair. This oil will fill in some of the cracks caused by the alkaline softening substance, and restore shine to your hair.

11. Brush, and style hair as desired.

Dry Hair in the Older Woman

The fourth and final major type of dry hair usually is first noted around middle age, when the hair starts turning gray. At this time, the body starts to lose its ability to produce pigment for the hair. As if to compensate for the loss of color, the body starts producing stronger, thicker hairs. Simultaneously, the scalp and the face produce less oil. The combination of less oil and increasing coarseness makes gray or graying hair stiff, wiry, and unmanageable. The control of these problems is approached in two steps:

1. The softening of coarse, thick hair.
2. The replacement of oil and water.

The shampoo should be plain and mild, such as those made for dry hair (e.g., BRECK FOR DRY HAIR). A plain cream rinse should be used at normal strength, and a light cream hairdressing should finish off each shampooing. To add water and oil to this type of hair, a monthly hot-oil treatment, employing a water-rich moisturizing lotion, can be very helpful.

A PROGRAM OF CARE FOR DRY HAIR
IN THE OLDER WOMAN

WEEKLY SHAMPOO

1. Wet your hair with water.

2. Pour on the shampoo and work it through the hair. Rinse out suds.

3. Repeat sudsing and rinsing.

4. Make up a cream rinse according to the manufacturer's instructions, using very warm water.

5. Pour the cream rinse on your hair and let it sit there for fifteen minutes.

6. Rinse out and blot off the extra moisture.

7. Dry your hair with or without setting it. Setting is not absolutely crucial to the appearance of the hair, as it is with coarse, curly hair. But, of course, it will look better if you set it.

8. When the hair has dried, rub a small dab of cream hairdressing between your hands and then rub your hands through your hair.

9. Brush, and arrange as desired.

The hot-oil treatment described in Chapter 15, pages 250–1, will work very well for gray hair, and should be given monthly for reconditioning.

Gray hair that has not been processed or dyed is not weak hair, and if any dandruff appears it can be treated with a sulfur shampoo. Use the dandruff shampoo in the place of the first sudsing and then proceed from there. If gray hair has been processed in any way, follow the program prescribed for the care of chemically treated hair, *not* the one for gray hair. The processing chemicals alter the normal structure of the hair and thus change the problems that arise in its natural state.

Dandruff

Dandruff is probably the most widespread hair problem. Whether your hair is short, curly, thick, or thin, dandruff can crop up and flake off.

It is basically a condition of *hyperkeratinization*, which means that the cells of the scalp are aging too rapidly into their hard, horny keratinized form. Normally, the body carefully controls the development of the cells of the scalp. These cells pass through stages of their development at an orderly rate, much as skin cells do. When they reach the scalp surface, and are completely dried out and dead, they fall off. Regular brushing and shampooing will remove these cells. Dandruff flakes will not appear. When the well-organized pattern of growth is disturbed, however, too many cells arrive at the surface in their dried form and become too numerous and too tightly packed to be removed by brushing and shampooing. These cells stick together and fall off in flakes; this condition is what we call dandruff.

Hyperkeratinization is responsible for dandruff in both dry and oily scalps. However, the *causes* of hyperkeratinization in oily scalps are very different from those causes operating in dry scalps.

Oily-scalp Dandruff

The sebaceous glands of an oily scalp produce too much oil. The *fatty acids* found in this natural oil irritate the scalp cells around the hair follicle. This irritation causes an increase in the growth of cells in the area and their rapid conversion to dried, dead, keratinized cells. The excess cells are the dandruff flakes.

To help this condition, it is necessary to slow down the scalp oil production and to use a thorough method of cleansing to remove the accumulation of dead cells and oil. Sulfur shampoos will do both jobs. Sulfur has a depressing effect on the activity of the oil glands and it also has the ability to break up the scalp dandruff scales. ENDEN, SEBULEX, SEBUTONE, and SELSUN are sulfur-containing dandruff shampoos. However, too frequent use of dandruff shampoos will make your scalp worse. They should only be used to bring the dandruff under control, not as a regular shampoo.

A DANDRUFF TREATMENT FOR OILY HAIR

1. Brush your hair well.

2. Wash your hair with a plain or lemon liquid shampoo for oily hair.

3. Use a dandruff (sulfur) shampoo as directed.

4. Rinse out with your regular shampoo.

5. Use a lemon rinse.

This treatment should replace your regular shampooing— no more than twice a week, however—until the dandruff is under control. Then use this treatment once every two weeks.

Dry-scalp Dandruff

A very dry scalp lacks water, not oil. This lack of water causes the excess flaking. The epidermis, as you will recall, is made up of cells with varying amounts of keratin. These cells must have water to maintain their strength and health. Without water, the cells are no longer held together and they fall away, as flakes of dandruff.

The treatment of dry-scalp dandruff aims at removing scales and restoring the oil-and-water balance to the scalp. To these ends, a mild dandruff shampoo containing zinc pyrothione (like HEAD & SHOULDERS) will do a good job of removing scales. A warm-oil treatment will feed water to the scalp and lay down a layer of oil, which will help retard the loss of water from the scalp due to evaporation.

A DANDRUFF TREATMENT FOR DRY HAIR

1. Brush your hair well with even strokes.

2. Heat one fourth cup or three tablespoons of lanolin lotion or cream. Spread on hair and work into your scalp.

3. Soak a towel in very hot water; wring it out; wrap it around your head and leave it there for twenty minutes.

4. Wash the oil out of your hair with a mild dandruff shampoo that contains zinc pyrothione. Sulfur is too harsh for dry hair.

5. Rinse head with lukewarm water.

Special Causes of Dandruff

DANDRUFF AND NORMAL SCALP: If you have dandruff and your scalp is neither extremely dry nor extremely oily, it is usually the result of inadequate care of the scalp. Insufficient brushing and superficial shampooing can lead to an accumulation of dead cells, and these will eventually flake off. Proper brushing and shampooing techniques will remove enough of these cells to keep the scalp smooth and clean. To clear up this dandruff use the following treatment. When the dandruff disappears, treat the hair with a regular program of hair care according to your hair type.

Instead of your usual shampoo, use the following program:

A DANDRUFF TREATMENT FOR MISMANAGED NORMAL HAIR

1. Brush your hair well, getting the bristles down close to the scalp.

2. Wet your hair, wash it once with plain shampoo.

3. Apply the aspirin rinse described below. Work it into your scalp for fifteen minutes.

4. Rinse out.

5. Apply the plain shampoo once again, and rinse out well.

ASPIRIN RINSE

Dissolve six aspirin tablets in a cup of warm water.
Pour over your hair, and work into the scalp.
Leave on for fifteen minutes and rinse thoroughly.

DANDRUFF AND TENSION: Many people notice that their dandruff becomes worse when they are tense, tired, or ill. All of these situations are similar in that they subject the body to what is called a stress situation.

Our natural body defenses are organized to protect essential functions such as breathing and blood circulation. In times of stress the body ignores the health of skin and hair, since their function is not essential to life. The balanced situation that enables the scalp to shed dead cells at a slow, even rate is disrupted and dandruff forms.

In addition, stress-caused changes in body chemistry affect oil production in the scalp. Tension in general will increase the amount of oil produced by the sebaceous glands, and the fatty acids in this oil will cause increased cell growth in the scalp. This kind of dandruff is best treated by following the program for oily-hair dandruff.

DANDRUFF AND PROCESSED HAIR: Processed (i.e., dyed, waved, or straightened) hair may also have dandruff problems. However, most of the effective dandruff treatments, such as the sulfur shampoos, are too strong for this type of hair. The sulfur will break up the hair molecules and cause the hair to mat and tangle. In some instances, whole sections of hair could mass together and form a lump of hair three to four inches wide that can be removed only by cutting away the matted hair. Dandruff in processed hair should be treated very gently, using a shampoo containing zinc pyrothione, a much milder yet still effective anti-dandruff agent.

A DANDRUFF TREATMENT FOR PROCESSED HAIR

1. Brush your hair gently; concentrate on the scalp, not on the hair.

2. Wet your hair; wash it once with a protein, acid-balanced shampoo such as AMINO-PON by Redken.

3. Use a mild dandruff shampoo that contains zinc pyrothione.

4. Rinse off.

5. Apply a protein cream rinse.

Note: Persistent dandruff that does not respond to any of the above treatments may be an indication of psoriasis, seborrhea, or other scalp disease that may require medical attention.

Thin and Thinning Hair

The one hair problem most people seem to worry about is hair loss and baldness. This is not surprising.

It is fairly easy to make oily hair less limp, frizzy hair smooth, and to cover over gray hair. But a receding hair line and/or a general thinning seems to be a continuous and irreversible process. This widely held concept is really not true. Many of the conditions that cause thinning of the hair can be easily managed.

"Skinny" Hair

The simplest cause of thin hair is "skinny" hair. The hair shaft itself is thin, often half as thin as the normal hair shaft. This does not indicate that anything is wrong with the hair itself. The thickness of the hair shaft, like the hair's color, is genetically determined. Skinny hair simply means that the genes determining hair thickness in your family were programmed for thin hair.

Blond hair is usually the skinniest type of hair, while red hair is usually the thickest. It takes approximately 140,000 blond hairs to provide a normal coverage of the scalp while only 90,000 red hairs are needed to create the same impression of hair fullness.

It is impossible to change the growth pattern of the hair follicles to naturally produce thicker hair shafts. It is possible, however, to artificially increase the diameter of the hair with hair dyes, special "body builders" for the hair, and protein conditioners.

Almost any kind of hair-coloring procedure will increase the diameter of the hair shaft. Permanent hair-coloring will enlarge the shaft because the high alkaline content in these mixtures swells the hair and ruffles up the outside of the cuticle, the outermost part of the hair shaft. The ruffling will make the hairs stand away from one another, giving an impression of additional fullness. Semi-permanent coloring will deposit a layer of dye on the outside of the hair shaft. This additional layer of substance on the surface of the hair shaft makes the hair seem thicker.

A group of products known as body builders for the hair are usually made up of a hair-spray-like solution, composed primarily of a resin or plastic that coats the hair with a layer of clear, quickly drying substance. This coating gives the hair shaft additional width because of the additional layers. As a result, the hairs look fuller.

There is nothing really magical about how these body builders work, but they do give a remarkable appearance of thicker hair. Most brands, by the way, are pretty much alike.

Hair products containing balsam also work on this principle. Balsam is a sticky resin that dries to a hard clear film, coating the hair shaft and increasing its diameter.

Protein shampoos and conditioners deposit a coating of proteins on the hair shaft, much like the coating of body builders.

If your hair has always been thin, if your hair has been blond or light brown in color, and if your hair texture has always been fine, skinny hair is probably your problem. Try a program of semi-permanent tints (in a shade close to your own if you do not wish to change the color of your hair), followed by use of protein shampoos and body-building conditioners.

Hair Breakage

The next cause of thin hair is the damage inflicted by too many permanents and too much bleaching. As with skinny hair, there is nothing wrong with the hair-growing apparatus. The problem here is really hair breakage. The chemicals from the permanenting and the repeated colorings have made the hair dry, brittle, and stiff. This type of hair cannot take the normal pressures of shampooing, brushing, or setting. The hairs break off at some point on the hair shaft, and frequently the break occurs near the roots. If many hairs are breaking off all over the head, the bulk of the hair will seem substantially reduced.

The bleaching, waving, and straightening of the hair do not affect the roots at all. The hair keeps growing, as evidenced by the constant need for retouching of the roots or redoing of the permanent. However, the more processing done to the hair, the worse the breakage will become.

To stop this breakage, the first step you should undertake is a three-month moratorium on all bleaching and waving. At the same time one should begin a concentrated program of acid shampoos to shrink and smooth the swollen, broken cuticle of the hair; protein conditioners to help strengthen the existing hair shaft; and warm-oil treatments to restore the moisture balance. A detailed step-by-step program for hair recovery will be found in Chapter 15, pages 238–40 and 249–52, those sections on the treatment of colored hair and permanented hair.

Skinny hair and broken hair are conditions in which external forces on the hair make it seem thinner, but the growth of the hair is not impaired. A situation where real hair growth is impaired occurs in the *brush-roller syndrome.*

Brush-roller Syndrome

Dermatologists recently began noticing increasing numbers of girls who appeared in their offices complaining that their hair was becoming very sparse. The doctors discovered that many of the patients frequently slept with rollers and clips in their hair. They spent an average of eight hours a day, one third of the entire day, with their hair tightly wound up and firmly positioned on the scalp.

The pressure of these rollers and clips against the scalp presumably cut down on the scalp's blood circulation. To maintain good health and growth, the hair shaft needs food and oxygen from the rich blood supply of the hair follicle. When this blood supply is drastically reduced (as by hair curlers and pins), the hair cannot get enough oxygen or food. The hair grows more slowly, and can even die from this imposed starvation. Because the scalp condition is so bad for growth, no new hair is encouraged to grow in and replace it, and since rollers are placed all over the head, this lack of circulation is present all over the scalp, thereby making the hair uniformly thin.

The cure is obvious: stop the constant use of rollers. Never sleep with rollers. Set your hair only after shampooing, not every night. When you do wash and set your hair, dry it with a hot-air dryer. The hair dries much faster this way, thus cutting down on the amount of time the hair is under tension on the rollers. Be sure to massage your hair well, and follow the basic shampoo/massage program outlined on pages 181–6.

It will take three to six months for new hair to grow in and be long enough to increase the volume of your hair. Take heart, for it definitely will grow.

Pony-tail Baldness

A closely related problem is called pony-tail baldness. This occurs in women who pull their hair back into a pony tail, or peruke, and hold it in place with a tightly bound rubber band. A hairstyle of this type puts tremendous pressure on the hair, especially at the hairline around the temples. The pressure cuts down the blood circulation on the scalp, and the same situation that occurred with the rollers and clips presents itself. However, in pony-tail baldness, the resulting thinning of the hair is limited to the area around the edges of the hair line, where the pressure is greatest.

To restore normal hair growth, the hair style must be changed. It is not necessary to cut your hair very short. Just be sure to stop pulling the hair straight back. It is not enough to replace rubber bands with wide barrettes. The hair should be allowed to hang free of all restraints. A normal program of shampoo/massage should be followed.

It is not wise to get a permanent, a straightening, or tinting done until the hair has filled out and filled in. These processes can weaken and break the hair, and the last thing you want at such times is additional breakage and hair loss.

Hair Loss Due to Tight Scalp

Impaired scalp circulation is also at the root of "tight scalp," a condition that can cause loss of hair. In this instance deposits of grease and dandruff have built up on the scalp to form a solid film that, in effect, strangles the blood circulation of the scalp. The condition is usually found in people with heavy dandruff problems and extremely oily hair. The control of tight scalp in these cases lies in the control of dandruff and oily hair; see pages 187–90 and 198–9 for complete instructions.

Tight scalp is also common in women who get their hair

"done" once a week or once every two weeks, and who try to maintain a coiffure between hairdressing appointments. They use gallons of hair spray to keep the hair rigid, and they lightly comb only the very top layers of the hair in order not to disturb the set. The grease and dandruff produced by the scalp is not disturbed for one or even two weeks. It coagulates into a solid mass that even the best shampoo cannot dislodge. The scalp is getting no stimulation whatsoever and the blood circulation is slowly being decreased by the mounting layer of grease and dandruff. Loss of hair soon follows.

Hair does not have to be washed more than once weekly, if it is dry or damaged hair. But it really should be brushed every day. You can switch to a style of hair that can survive daily brushing. This usually means either no teasing or choosing a shorter hair style.

If this is impossible, buy an electric vibrator and give your scalp a good rub with it each day. The vibrator will not dislodge the layer of grease and dirt. But it will stimulate the scalp's blood circulation and decrease the hair loss.

At the weekly shampoo, use a rubber shampoo brush to dislodge the oily dandruff layer. Have the hairdresser give your scalp a really good massage; your scalp should feel warm and tingly from the increased blood circulation.

Hair Loss in Pregnancy

Hair fall in pregnancy is extremely common. Under normal conditions, the hair cycle is regulated by an internal time clock in the follicle. At a certain point in time, the hair in the follicle dies, and a new hair begins to grow in its place. After a while, the dead hair falls out or is pulled out. It is soon replaced by a new hair and its loss is never noticed. Each hair dies at a different time, so that the death and regrowth of the hair is never noticed. The hair population of the head seems stable.

During pregnancy, the hair growth pattern is changed. Much of the body's energy is directed to maintaining vital functions in the mother. The body now "feels" that hair growth is not "essential" to survival. So when a hair dies on schedule, no new hair starts to grow to take its place. As the pregnancy progresses, more hairs die off and are not replaced. The bulk of the hair gets thinner. By the time the baby is born, enough hair has fallen and not been replaced to produce sparse areas on the scalp. It takes about three months after giving birth to get the hair growing in its regular cycle.

In some women, hair loss does not occur during pregnancy, but only after delivery. This is because the hair that died during pregnancy remained in the follicle and did not fall out. After the baby is born, the body starts producing new hairs in the scalp. This is a signal for all the dead hairs to fall out. When they do, the volume of hair decreases noticeably. It will take up to six months for enough new hairs to grow in to make up for the hair loss.

Not much can be done to stimulate the hair follicle during pregnancy. Some doctors feel that a lack of iron might be a contributing factor. Iron pills and the good diet prescribed by your obstetrician can control iron deficiency, and under normal circumstances should be adequate to control any hair problem due to iron deficiency.

While the hair is thin, use body builders and protein conditioners that have already been described for skinny hair. These do not make the hair grow any better, but they do make the existing hairs seem thicker.

Good scalp and hair hygiene is essential during pregnancy. It will stand the hair in good stead when it resumes normal growth after delivery. Good care consists of a careful program of the proper kinds of shampoo, rinses, massage, and brushing.

Hair Loss Due to Poor Health

Overwork, long illnesses such as hepatitis or mononucleosis, a heart attack, major surgery, or even serious mental strain can produce a debilitated physical condition frequently accompanied by hair loss. The causes are very similar to those of pregnancy hair loss. The body is throwing all of its vital energies into keeping more essential functions going. It has no energy to spare for starting new hair growth.

To stop this kind of hair thinning, the underlying medical problem has to be resolved. Plenty of rest, a high protein diet, adequate medical or psychiatric care should strengthen the body and renew its interest in growing your hair.

While the subject of diet is being raised, it is interesting to note that some hair loss problems have been traced to crash diets, macrobiotic diets, and vegetarian regimens, all of which are often very low in essential proteins and vitamins.

In *kwashiorkor*, a disease associated with severe malnutrition, one of the characteristic findings is loss of hair, with complete arrest of hair growth. The hair color also changes from its original shade to a reddish blond, indicating the body's inability to synthesize the hair pigments.

Without sufficient proteins the body loses its stores of raw materials, which are necessary for growth and repair. Since the hair is one of the most rapidly growing parts of the body, it is very sensitive to this reduction in basic body materials. In addition, the body usually channels its resources to the essential life services, so that the hair is left unsupplied. Without the basic proteins, the hair does not grow. Old hairs die and are not replaced.

A diet sufficiently high in protein will avoid this problem. It has been estimated that a good diet consists of one half gram of protein for each pound of body weight in order to maintain good nutrition. Look at the table of protein values below and see how many grams you are getting each day.

A TABLE OF PROTEIN VALUES

PROTEIN-RICH FOODS

FOOD	GRAMS OF PROTEIN
1 cup of whole or skimmed milk	9
1 oz. hard cheese	8
1 cup of yogurt	8
1 egg	6
1 cup of cottage cheese	34
3 oz. hamburger (or other red meat)	23
3 oz. broiled chicken	20
3 oz. canned clams	7
3 oz. broiled swordfish (similar for other fish steaks)	24
3 oz. broiled shrimp	21
1 tablespoon of peanut butter	4
3 oz. roast lamb	20

3 oz. roast pork	**20**
3 oz. roast veal	**23**

All the previous cases of thinning hair have been relatively easy to understand and control. Now we are going to deal with a more frightening kind of hair fall, *alopecia areata.*

Alopecia Areata

This condition begins with the sudden appearance of a coin-shaped patch of totally bald scalp.

The hair has fallen out of this area very quickly. In two days a previously normal area of scalp can display a round, hairless patch. There can be more than one bald patch on the scalp, and if they overlap, they can form large hairless areas.

The exact causes of this hair problem are hard to trace. There is no single cause, although a number of cases have been traced to severe emotional problems. A particularly trying episode in one's life, the death of a friend or family member, a drastic change in lifestyle (e.g., marriage or divorce)—emotional strains such as these have been associated with the appearance of bald spots.

An accident or blow to the head has also been shown to precipitate alopecia areata. So too can an underactive thyroid, pregnancy, and the beginning of menopause.

As frightening as bald patches might look, and as vague as the understanding of their causes may seem, alopecia areata is basically self-limiting. The hair usually grows back by itself quickly, after a relatively short period of time. In some cases, where the area of hair fall has been extensive, cortisone pills have been prescribed by dermatologists in order to encourage hair growth. This treatment has met with good success, but its use is limited only to severe cases. Time and patience will usually be medicine enough, and healthy new hair should fill in the bald spots in about three months.

Massage and hair tonics are not advisable to stimulate hair growth in alopecia areata. In a desperate attempt to get their hair to grow back, many people can injure their bald spots with too enthusiastic treatments. Just maintain good scalp hygiene, refrain from further hair processing, and the whole episode will soon be forgotten. If you worry too much about them, your bald spots can be aggravated by your understandable anxiety.

Hair Loss After Menopause

As a woman grows older her body grows more slowly. The cells do not reproduce as quickly as before. The slowing-down processes also affect the growth of hair. When the hairs die off and fall out, it takes quite a while for the new hair to replace them. At the same time, the blood circulation is substantially decreased. This also adds to the general decline in the growth of hair.

With the hair falling out faster than it can be replaced, the hair begins to look sparse. It can also become brittle and dry and break off more easily.

Scalp massage can go a long way in giving the circulation a much-needed boost, thereby helping the hair growth cycle. Conditioning with water-rich creams, protein rinses, and acid-based shampoos can give flexibility and bounce to thin, aging hair and make it seem thicker. Follow the same massage and conditioning programs prescribed for damaged hair.

Male-pattern Baldness

The last cause of thinning hair is something called Male-pattern Baldness (MPB for short). This is the most common cause of hair loss for men, affecting about 60 percent of the adult male population sometime in their lives. It consists of thinning hair at the temples, the front hair line, and the crown of the head. This thinning progresses until the entire top of the head is bald, leaving only a fringe around the ears and at the nape of the neck.

Mercifully, this is very rare in women. When it does occur it generally indicates an abnormal hormonal condition similar to that involved with the growth of excess facial hair. (See Chapter 9, pages 139–47.) MPB in women is frequently accompanied by an increase of facial and body hair, a change in the menstrual cycle, and a flare-up of severe acne. This problem is something to be handled only by a highly trained doctor.

Most of the time, once the underlying cause is found the

patient responds well to treatment. Her scalp hair will grow in, the unwanted facial and body hair falls out, the skin clears up, and all is back to normal. As mentioned before, this is a fairly rare situation, but it is something to keep in mind when considering hair fall problems.

14 / Special Hair Problems

Gray Hair

Most "gray" hair is usually not really gray in color, but a mixture of white hairs among the normal shades of brown, blond, red, or black. White hair is due to a lack of melanin granules in the cortex of the hair shaft. Usually occurring with advancing age, this lack of melanin granules means the body is losing its ability to synthesize the pigments from enzymes and proteins.

True gray hairs are quite rare. They are caused by a decrease (not a total absence) in the pigment content in the hair shaft. The visual mixing of pigmented and nonpigmented areas of hair is seen as gray color.

Dark hair does not really gray earlier than other colors. It is the striking contrast between the white and dark hair that makes the hair seem more obviously gray.

Most people start to sprout a few gray hairs at about thirty, and become progressively grayer over the next twenty years. More and more of their hairs lack pigment. At around sixty or seventy the hair often turns completely white, which means that all the hairs on the head have lost their pigment granules.

Sometimes hair starts turning gray prematurely, in the early twenties. This may often be the result of genetic factors, since the tendency seems to run in families. Severe stress, mental illness, serious physical ailments, and traumatic experiences have been associated with both premature gray hair and the acceleration of graying. The *why* of this phenomenon is not known.

Gray Hair and Vitamins

Much has been written on the relationship of vitamins to gray hair. Laboratory studies on animals have shown that certain B vitamins, such as biotin and pantothenic acid, will reduce grayness. But animals have a very different hair growth cycle from human beings, and attempts to repeat these results in people (either with creams or pills) have not been very successful unless the persons are truly deficient in B vitamins. However, deficiency of B vitamins in otherwise healthy Americans is a medical rarity. It is usually seen among alcoholics who eat only minimally, persons with severe debilitating intestinal disease, and persons who for one reason or another do not or cannot eat. Gray hair is usually a minor feature of this deficiency problem, for in addition the person suffers from neurological symptoms (i.e., tingling and numbness in the feet) and severe anemia. While biotin is highly touted as a cure-all for many skin and hair problems, it is a very commonly found vitamin and there are very few documented cases of biotin deficiency in the medical literature. It has been shown, however, that raw egg white can interfere with the activity of biotin in the body. One of the few cases involved an Italian baker who existed for years on a diet consisting of nothing but twelve raw eggs and two bottles of red wine a day. Living on the bizarre diet, he finally showed biotin deficiency symptoms. This case gives you an idea as to how outlandish a diet must be before real biotin deficiency problems appear.

If you have gray hair, go ahead and try taking vitamin B complex supplements. You may be one of the two to three percent of persons who respond. Vitamin B is probably most effective for persons whose grayness began after a severe strain, such as a long debilitating illness or a harrowing emotional experience. This is not surprising, since such strains would deplete the health maintenance reserves of the body and vitamins may be more in demand at such a time.

What Can Be Done for Gray Hair

Once hair has started turning gray, there is nothing presently known that can be done to reverse this process. There are, however, many hair dyes designed specifically to color gray hair (see Chapter 15, "Processed Hair"). Or, if you are all gray and do not wish to change back to your original color, there are many things you can do to make gray hair more attractive.

The most common complaint about gray hair is that it takes on a yellowish tinge. This discoloring results from a host of factors: tobacco smoke, carbolic acid (found in dry, powder, shampoos), setting lotions, and especially dandruff shampoos containing resorcinol.

Examination of some yellowish gray hairs under the microscope, however, does reveal a diffuse yellow pigment inside the hair shaft, apparently another manifestation of the aging-related changes in melanin production. The easiest way to get rid of this yellow tinge, the result of either external or internal factors, is to treat the hair with a bluing rinse.

TO PREPARE BLUING RINSE

1. Add one tablespoonful of laundry bluing to a quart of warm water.

2. After shampooing your hair, blot it dry with a towel.

3. Pour the dilute bluing solution onto your hair (covering your eyes) and let set for ten minutes.

4. Rinse out with lukewarm water.

As hair gets grayer, it also seems to get stronger. It is as though the body is putting all of its power into the thickness and resiliency of the hair after it loses its color. It also gets dryer and coarser. This change has nothing to do with graying hair, but accompanies the general aging process.

People who had fine, oily hair will notice that their hair becomes drier and more unruly. It is wise to alter hair care programs at this time to take into account these changes in hair texture. Sometimes only a cream rinse is needed to bring your hair into line. If your hair is now tougher and coarser, you should change to a shampoo for dry hair and start moisturizing conditioners and monthly warm-oil treatments.

A PROGRAM OF CARE FOR DRY, COARSE, GRAY HAIR

AT YOUR WEEKLY SHAMPOO

1. Brush hair.

2. Massage scalp.

3. Wet hair, add shampoo for dry hair.

4. Work in, rinse out, repeat.

5. Twice monthly, use a bluing rinse (see page 214).

6. Use a cream conditioner for dry hair (like TAME by Toni).

7. Rinse out.

8. Blot dry gently.

9. Comb through and set. Do not use setting lotions or hair sprays. They have a tendency to turn gray hair yellow.

Baby-fine Hair

Fine, slippery hair always hangs board straight. It has a wonderful sheen immediately after shampooing but quickly becomes lank, dull, and oily. It seems unable to take a set, and certainly does not seem to hold one. It is often light-brown or blond hair, and only rarely red or black.

The situation is complicated. First of all, this hair is usually thin hair. There are simply not that many hairs per square inch of scalp as are found on, say, black, curly hair. The hairs themselves are probably narrower in diameter than other types of hair.

The second problem with fine hair is that when it becomes oily, it sticks together, making the coiffure flatter and thinner than ever.

The last problem, and the most important, is that the cuticles of these hairs are very tight and smooth. Ordinarily, this is a desirable state for a hair to be in and it would usually increase the beauty of the hair. The mirror-like sheen of fine, slippery hair is an indication of its remarkably smooth cuticle.

The cuticle is so tight and so smooth that nothing can penetrate it. Water cannot get inside to break the protein bonds to let the hair rearrange itself during setting. The absence of little cracks in the cuticle makes it impossible for the hairs to lock into one another, forming a distinct line of coiffure. This kind of hair is often termed "virgin hair." It has never had any processing done to it, and the cuticle is totally "unviolated."

Help for Baby-fine Hair

To give this hair body, bounce, and form, a three-pronged approach should be used:

1. The oiliness should be controlled.

2. The diameter of the hair should be built up with protein conditioners.

3. The cuticle should be roughed up by mild processing (either tinting or waving).

The oiliness can be taken care of as described in the section on oily hair in Chapter 13, omitting the acid rinse at the end of the shampoo (pages 187–9).

The diameter of the hair can be gradually increased with the constant use of protein-based shampoos and conditioners. The dissolved proteins in these products lay down a layer of amino acids welcomed by the hair shaft itself. Successive protein treatments will increase this layer of protein on the hair, and up to a point increase its diameter. It is like adding layers in a sandwich; the more pieces of meat, cheese, or bread you add, the thicker the sandwich becomes.

Strange as it may seem, since in so many hair problems we are constantly trying to smooth and tighten the cuticle, the best treatment for slippery hair is to rough up the cuticle with alkaline rinses or processing (such as permanent-waving or coloring).

At first glance, permanent-waving would seem to be the best answer: it gives body to the hair as well as helping it to hold a set. There are drawbacks, however. Slippery hair is very resistant to waving solutions. After several unsuccessful attempts to get such hair to take a wave, one is tempted to leave the waving solution on too long. The result is a frizzy, dry, drab mess. It is a very small step for this kind of hair from no wave to the "Harpo Marx look." Permanent-waving is usually not the answer for fine, slippery hair.

Coloring is a better solution. It will also rough up the cuticle and help the hair behave, and it is much easier to control the strength and the effects of your coloring solutions. This coloring will also add highlights and rich, deep tones to hair that is often dull and vaguely colored. Even a simple ammonia-peroxide-soap solution rinsed onto the hair will be alkaline enough to cause cuts in the hair cuticle and thereby make the hair hold and set better.

To color the hair, you can use a shampoo-in color, a one-step tint, or section-frosting. With proper conditioning, thin, slippery hair can enjoy just about the best results that coloring has to offer because it thrives on the alkaline substances contained in hair dyes.

See the next chapter for a complete discussion of the different dyes and techniques that go into using them.

ROUGHING UP THE HAIR CUTICLE
WITHOUT DYES OR TINTS

EVERY SIX WEEKS

1. Wash your hair as usual.

2. Blot dry.

3. Do not use herb rinses or a protein pack.

4. Make up a solution of: 1 tablespoon glycerin; 1 tablespoon shampoo; 1 tablespoon ammonia; and 1 cup water. Shake this combination well.

5. Massage into the hair; be sure to get the ends covered.

6. Let sit for ten minutes.

7. Rinse out with cool water.

8. Blot dry.

9. Set without setting lotion.

Hair and the Sun

Hair and skin are made up of basically the same substance, a protein called keratin. Since they are similarly composed they share many of the same properties. They both need water to remain soft and flexible; they both thrive on acidic-based cosmetic aids; they both use oil as a shield against water evaporation; and, finally, both hair and skin suffer damage from excess sun.

Sun-damaged hair is stiff, dry, and dull. The ends are frayed and the hair is very difficult to set and style. The hair becomes so dry and brittle that it breaks off and seems thin and sparse.

The sun can also change the color of your hair. It will give red-orange highlights to natural brown and black hair, and it will lighten naturally blond hair. In all fairness, it must be said that some of these color changes are attractive; however, the concurrent damage to the hair itself makes sunbleaching not too practical.

Strong sunlight can wreak havoc with tinted hair color, bringing out greenish or brassy tones. Tinted hair, permanented hair, and straightened hair will suffer greater damage than virgin or unprocessed hair.

Even a small amount of sun delivers a one-two punch to processed hair. The first effect of the sun is *dehydration*. The sun's heat evaporates a great deal of the moisture present in the hair shaft. Lack of water makes the keratin, already weakened by processing, brittle and inflexible. Noticeable dehydration can occur even after only a few hours of exposure to the sun. However, if the hair is given a chance to rest, out of the sun, the water content will return to its normal level within a few days, and the hair will recover its former softness.

Unfortunately, most people spend more than one day in the sun at a time, and the water level does not have a chance to return to its normal level in a natural way. Continued exposure to the sun will cause additional and irreversible damage to processed hair. The dehydration of the hair gets worse and worse with each hour of exposure to the sun. The keratin becomes so weak and brittle from lack of water that it crumbles. When this occurs, the hair becomes fragile and breaks off easily. It has been so badly damaged that, without reconditioning, it cannot return to a normal state by itself.

The second punch of the sun's attack on processed hair is the bleaching effect. The sun will change the chemistry of the hair dyes, often destroying a carefully chosen color. It will fade the artificial color, or produce a green and metallic sheen in the hair. By changing the color it will make reapplication of new tint complicated. The roots will have to be changed to the originally chosen shade and then the rest of the head will have to be recolored to blend in with the roots.

All sun-damaged hair is weak, unhealthy hair. It is often too weak to be colored, permanented, or straightened. Such processing puts a strain on the hair, and this strain on already weakened hair can result in a horrifying loss of hair. At the same time, even moderately sun-damaged hair will give poor results with processing. The hair will absorb the dye unevenly, producing splotchy coloration. It also has a tendency to become very frizzy after permanenting, and stiff and rigid after straightening.

As bad as all of this sounds, sun damage to hair is much less serious than it is to skin. The hair can be repaired to a great extent by protein conditioners and moisturizing creams. In severe cases, where flexibility and shine are impossible to restore, the new growth of hair will come in healthy and undamaged.

Preventing sun damage to the hair is ridiculously simple. Wear a hat or scarf on the head when in the sun. Anyone with processed hair should be sure to keep her head covered from the sun. Unprocessed hair can safely take short periods of exposure to sun, one to two hours a day. During any real exposure to sun, such as on the beach or on a boat, the head should be covered.

The treatment of sunburned hair is very similar to the treatment of hair damaged by processing. Reconditioners designed to improve the water balance of the hair will restore elasticity and flexibility. A nonalkaline shampoo will encourage the keratin to firm up. A protein conditioner will fill in the cracks in the outer layers of the hair, making each strand stronger and shinier, and a hot-oil treatment will feed water to thirsty, dried-out hair and help it keep this water in, until the hair is healthy enough to maintain its own water balance.

A RECONDITIONING TREATMENT FOR SUN-DAMAGED HAIR

1. Wet hair with warm water. Do not shampoo.

2. Heat one fourth cup of lanolin-rich lotion (lanolin is closest to natural hair oil) in a small saucepan until it is hot to the touch (not simmering). *Caution:* If oil is too hot, scalp burns and permanent hair loss may result.

3. Dip a two-inch paint brush into the hot oil and "paint it" all over the head, forcing it down to the scalp. Do not concentrate on the scalp, however: this treatment is mainly for the hair.

4. When the whole head is covered, and all the oil is used up, wrap the head in SARAN WRAP. Put on a heating cap if you have one and turn it to medium heat.

5. Let your head "cook" for twenty to thirty minutes.

6. Remove the headgear.

7. Wash your hair once or twice with a protein-acid shampoo.

8. Use a protein conditioner; then rinse and blot dry.

Split Ends

Split ends, those ragged tips of the hair, are an indication of the damage done to the keratin of the hair shaft.

Sometimes, this damage indicates that the keratin has lost too much water and is crumbling. On the other hand, this damage may be mechanical, as from the stresses generated by brushes, hair rollers, and bobby pins. The keratin is weaker when wet, and crushing the hair shafts with pin curls or on brush rollers will break the hair and result in split ends. Finally, cold-waved or colored hair will also show split ends, part of the more general disintegration of heavily processed hair. The care of this type of hair problem is discussed in the next chapter.

Simply cutting off these split ends is not the whole answer. The new ends of the cut hair will soon start to fray. One must try to rebuild the keratin in the whole hair shaft in order to stop the hair from splitting. You must try to build up the keratin with protein shampoos and conditioners; to tighten the keratin with an acid rinse; and to lock the water into the hair shaft with special cream conditioners.

The following techniques will strengthen the whole hair shaft. Do not cut off split ends before treatments. Wait and see if the protein program will repair the damage. If it is too late for the split ends, and they still remain frayed and frazzled, they should be cut off. But now the rest of the hair will not fray again because of the treatment.

A PROGRAM OF CARE FOR SPLIT ENDS

1. Brush hair carefully to remove loose dust and flakes.

2. Wet hair and pour on protein shampoo (AMINO-PON by Redken or PROTEIN 21 by Mennen are excellent brands). Work the shampoo into your hair and rinse.

3. Repeat the sudsing, and rinse again.

4. Apply a protein conditioner (such as PROTEIN 21 CONDI-TIONER or P.P.T. 77 by Redken). If your hair is oily, pour conditioner on the lower lengths of hair. Do *not* use conditioner near the scalp.

5. It will take about a month of twice-weekly treatments to correct a split-end condition. This treatment should thereafter be repeated once each month to keep the hair strong and tight.

SOME DO'S AND DON'T'S

1. Pin curls promote split ends. Try to wrap each section of hair in an end paper before twisting the hair and fastening it with a clip or bobby pin. This will reduce the pressure of the metal clip on the hair.

2. Use end papers on your hair when you roll your hair on the rollers.

3. Plastic brushes and combs with broken teeth can catch the hair and crack its keratin. Be sure to use a comb whose teeth are uniformly spaced throughout its width. It is extremely important if you have split ends to avoid a very fine comb, because it can cause excessive friction on the hair and make your split ends worse.

The bristles of the brush should be firm and well spaced, and it is important for split ends that it should be graded so the longest bristles are in the center of the brush.

4. Never jerk a comb or brush through the hair. They should be drawn smoothly and gently through the hair. When the hair is long use the following method to avoid snapping the ends: The comb or the brush should be drawn through lengths of about six inches at a time. That is, first brush the hair around the crown, then hold the hair at ear level and pull the comb or brush from this point to your shoulders. Continue in this way, brushing six inches of hair at a time.

. . .

Dull Hair

There are four basic factors most often responsible for dull hair: processing, oiliness, hard water, and melanin content.

Processing

Heavily processed hair—for example, hair that has been cold-waved or bleached—results in the cracking and drying of the hair shaft. To be shiny, the cuticle, the outermost layer of the hair shaft, must be smooth and uncracked.

Processing cracks the cuticle by actually eating away the keratin coating of the hair shaft. It also leaches out water from the hair shaft, which further damages the cuticle. To make this hair shiny again, the keratin must be rebuilt and the cracks closed. This is done by using protein shampoos and rinses, which build up the keratin layer, as well as by using acidifying treatments, which close up the cracks. For a complete guide to the care of processed hair, see Chapter 15.

Oiliness

Dull hair can also arise from oily, greasy hair. Some oil, of course, is necessary to give the hair its nice sheen. Oil also fills in the tiny cracks in the cuticle. Clean, fresh oil makes a smooth, slick film on the surface of each hair, which reflects light evenly. This same oil, if allowed to remain for too long a period, will attract dust and dirt. These particles of dirt deposited on the hair shaft make the shaft's surface uneven and bumpy. The natural oil, which is colorless when it comes out of the follicle, becomes a cloudy gray after it is exposed to the air, which makes the hair even duller.

Oil-dulled hair is best treated by controlling the basic oiliness. For details on the management of this problem, see pages 187–90 on the care of oily hair.

· · ·

Hard Water

Soap residues can leave a dulling film on otherwise well-conditioned hair. This may result from insufficient rinsing after shampoo. But even with the most vigorous rinsing, soap can sometimes remain on the hair. This occurs because of the chemical reaction of hard (calcium-containing) water with soap in your shampoo. This reaction deposits a rough mixture of mineral salts and soap on your hair, making it dull and lifeless. Hard water exists in most areas of the country; in fact, just about every area fifty miles inland from the sea is a hard-water area.

If you live inland, and have normal or oily hair (unprocessed), and take relatively good care of your hair and scalp, but nevertheless have a dull look to your hair, it could be due to the hard water you are using to clean your hair. This problem can be very easily overcome by using a strong lemon rinse at the end of each shampoo.

LOW-COST HOMEMADE PREPARATIONS FOR USE IN HARD-WATER AREAS

A HARD-WATER LEMON RINSE FOR BLONDES

1. Squeeze out the juice of two lemons.

2. Add two cups of water to lemon juice.

3. Pour this lemon–water mixture over your hair following the final shampooing. Work into your hair and scalp.

4. Let it sit for five minutes and rinse out with lukewarm water.

A HARD-WATER RINSE FOR DARK HAIR

1. Squeeze out the juice of one lemon and strain it.

2. Add one cup of cool tea (any brand will do).

3. Pour the tea-lemon mixture over your head following the final shampooing. Work into your hair and scalp.

4. Let it sit for five minutes and rinse out with cool water.

A HARD-WATER RINSE FOR DRY HAIR (ALL COLORS)

1. Combine one cup cool water with one teaspoon apple-cider vinegar.

2. Pour this mixture over your hair following the final shampooing. Work into your hair and scalp.

3. Let it sit for five minutes and rinse out with lukewarm water.

Melanin Content

The last and most difficult problem causing dull hair concerns the color of the hair itself. This problem usually affects people with dark-blond to medium-brown hair. These hair shades are based on a combination of black, red, and blond melanin pigment granules. Like any mixed color, the evenness and brightness of the shades depend on the amounts of the different pigments that make up the hair color. Some combinations give a rich, warm, honey-brown tone, while others produce a murky, grayish-brown tone.

There is nothing that can be done to make the body produce different kinds of melanin. However, the color of your hair can easily be enriched or changed with artificial coloring. For the best way to choose your color highlighting agent and the techniques to use, see the section on hair coloring in Chapter 15.

Dull hair resulting from poor color is frequent among blondes and red-haired women when they reach their forties and fifties. The bright natural colors of the hair seem pale and faded, because of the white hairs mixed with the natural colors. In a woman with dark hair, these white hairs are distinctly visible and give the hair a mottled gray appearance. But in fair-haired women, there is not such a contrast in color tone, and the white hairs only dilute the natural color. Think of mixing paints. If you add white paint to a bright red color, you will get a paler red color.

Faded color can be brightened with artificial tints. It is difficult to pick exactly the right color in this situation, and the choice is best left to an experienced beautician.

15 / Processed Hair

Hair Coloring

If you're 5'1" and want to be 5'8", it's too bad. If you've got brown eyes and want to have pale-gray eyes, forget it. But if you're a brunette and dream of having red hair, you're in luck. Hair coloring is the easiest feature to change or improve. Properly done, and properly conditioned, tinted or dyed hair can look far better than your natural hair color. It is relatively inexpensive, 95 percent safe, and most often it is easy to do. To obtain the best results, however, it is absolutely vital to understand the different dyes and what they do to your hair.

Color Rinses and Highlighting Shampoos

The simplest and most temporary hair coloring is provided by the color rinses and the highlighting shampoos. The coloring agents of both products are called *certified colors*. Each batch of certified color is tested for safety by the F.D.A. These dyes are readily washed out. Color rinses are frequently available in an inexpensive powdered form. They can darken blond hair to red, brown, or black shades. For dark shades of hair, however, these temporary colors can only add highlight. The effects tend to be uneven, especially when you are going from blond hair to red or black hair. The color can streak, and it comes out with combing.

Color shampoos are designed to bring out the highlights of natural hair color. They are not really meant to change hair color. Helena Rubinstein puts out a line of these products. A person with medium-brown hair can use the blond-toned shampoo for blond tones; the brown shampoo to enrich brown coloring; the red shampoo for red shadings; and the black to darken the hair to a deeper brown. But using the black shampoo on blond hair will produce only a muddy brown color. These changes are very slight and short-lived.

Semi-permanent Tinting Agents

Semi-permanent dyes can highlight and enrich the natural color of the hair; enhance the appearance of gray hair without changing its grayness; and cover, or blend gray hair in to bring back original color. They cannot make dark hair light, and should not be used to try to completely change the color of your hair. If used for this purpose, they produce a streaky, uneven color with much of the original hair color showing through. You should pick a color one or two shades lighter or darker than your own natural color to get the best results.

To blend in gray hair, choose a color one shade lighter or the same shade as your own hair. To cover gray hair, use a color one shade darker than your own.

LOVING CARE by Clairol is an example of such a product.

CARE OF HAIR TREATED WITH SEMI-PERMANENT TINTS: Semi-permanent tints do not contain any peroxide, ammonia, or other chemicals that can break up or soften keratin. Under these circumstances, protein shampoos and conditioners are not necessary. However, the alkaline pH of the tint may do some damage to your hair, so be certain that the shampoo you use is acidic (like AMINO-PON).

Permanent Hair-coloring Products

Permanent hair-coloring products contain vegetable, metallic, or aniline dyes. The most popular type used today is the aniline dye. Vegetable and metallic dyes are rarely used professionally because of their poor cosmetic results and their bad effect on the hair. These dyes are still available, however, for home use.

VEGETABLE DYES: These deposit a coating of dye on the cuticle of the hair shaft. Henna, a red tint, is the most commonly used vegetable dye today. Application of henna is a very messy, tedious procedure. It provides a poor-quality color. Repeated use causes a buildup of color, which leads to orange overtones. Henna can make the hair dry and stiff. Hennaed hair does not take well to permanent-waving, straightening, or coloring with semi-permanent or aniline dyes.

METALLIC DYES: These, also called *color restorers*, are the progressive type of dye. They are combed through the hair, and after several days gradually cover gray hairs. They act by depositing a coating of dye on your hair. The dye produces a dark, flat, unnatural color with no highlights. The hair feels dry and stiff. The colors usually fade into strange-looking tones: metallic dyes containing silver develop a greenish hue; those with copper, a reddish glow; and the lead dyes create a purple cast. Hair dyed with metallic products will not react well to waving, straightening, or to any other type of hair coloring.

Before any major processing (such as permanent-waving or coloring) can be done to hair treated with metallic dyes or vegetable dyes, these dyes must be removed. There are preparations such as METALEX by Clairol, which will gradually remove the dyes without changing the natural color of the hair.

A PROCEDURE FOR REMOVING VEGETABLE AND METALLIC DYES

1. Spray METALEX full strength onto the hair. Two ounces (a fourth of a cup) is enough.

2. Saturate the hair thoroughly with the solution. Be sure to get it all over the entire hair strand, from the roots to the tips of the hair.

3. Work this solution into your hair, but *not* into the scalp. Pile hair on top of head and wrap it in SARAN WRAP.

4. Fit a heating cap, or wrap a hot, damp, but not wet towel

on for a total of thirty minutes. When the towel cools replace it with a new hot one.

5. After thirty minutes, rinse thoroughly with warm water. Shampoo with mild soap. Do not color your hair immediately. This procedure may have to be repeated several times before the metallic and/or the vegetable dyes have been removed. You can tell when the dyes are gone when your hair is close to its natural color.

Use the METALEX or a similar product twice a week until the dyes seem to have disappeared. Wait three or four days before you recolor, then try a test strand to see if your hair has recovered from those bad dyes and can now successfully take an aniline dye or semi-permanent dye. If the test strand takes the dye well, color the rest of the hair. If not, try a few more treatments, and then test another strand of hair. Sometimes the hair is so badly damaged from vegetable and metallic dyes that one must wait for it to grow out and be cut off before any more processing can be done to the hair.

ANILINE DYES: These are by far the most satisfactory type of permanent hair coloring. Originally discovered in Germany in 1893, they have been modified and improved so that sixty thousand different shades are now available.

The way aniline derivative dyes give color to your hair is extraordinary (see Diagram 27).

The molecules of the dye are tiny and colorless. The colorless dye is mixed with a developer, generally peroxide, and quickly

Diagram 27.   HOW ANILINE DYE WORKS ON HAIR

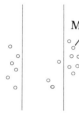
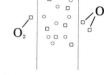
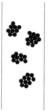

Molecules of Dye

Molecules of Dye
Going into Hair Shaft

Oxygen Introduced
into Hair

In the Presence
of Oxygen, Molecules
of Dye Combining
and Developing Color

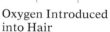

○ Molecule of Dye   □ Oxygen (O_2)   • Molecule of Developed Dye

applied to the hair. At first the molecules of the dye are so tiny that they are small enough to get into the hair shaft, through the cuticle, where they settle in the cortex. Once there, they begin to react with the oxygen molecules produced by the peroxide. This chemical reaction stimulates the molecules of the aniline dye to combine with one another; and by combining, the molecules develop the color your hair will ultimately adopt. Scientists have been able to make thousands of different colors by changing and switching the arrangements of molecules in the basic aniline dye.

The colored molecules are permanently stuck in the hair shaft because by combining they have grown too big to get out from within the cuticle. Shampooing cannot dislodge them as it can the colors of temporary or semi-permanent rinses.

Any chemical reaction as complex as this is going to create some problems. About 10 percent of the people who use these products will develop an allergy to them and break out in red splotches. For this reason, a sensitivity test must be performed on *every* person *each* time an aniline product is used. Even if you are not allergic to aniline dyes, these should never be used anywhere around the eyes.

And if someone is allergic, and the dyes are used in areas around the eyes, on the eyebrows or the eyelashes, blindness can result as a consequence of the severe allergic reaction that follows.

Eyelash and eyebrow dyes are forbidden by federal (F.D.A.) law to contain aniline dyes or derivatives. While commercial distribution is technically outlawed, small quantities of these products have been brought back by travelers or have found their way into private beauty salons. Therefore, carefully read the label of any lash and brow dye you want to try.

All manufacturers of hair-coloring products containing aniline dyes provide instructions for performing a *patch test*. A patch test of hair dye must be done at least twenty-four hours before coloring the hair. If you are sensitive to this particular dye the allergic reaction has time to develop. It will only appear at the site of the patch test. This protects you from developing a truly bad allergic reaction when you actually color your hair.

A patch test is performed at two spots: behind the ear and at the crook of the elbow. Before testing, wash both areas with mild soap and water, and pat dry. Dip a cotton swab into the dye solution and apply to the test areas. The solution should be exactly the same as the one you hope to apply to your hair. If you use a semi-permanent tint you simply dip the cotton swab into the bottle of dye. If it is a permanent color you must pour out a teaspoon of the dye and a teaspoon of the developer, mix them, and apply the mixture to the test areas.

Examine the patch test twenty-four hours later. If the skin is perfectly clear, you can go ahead with hair coloring. If there is even the slightest bit of redness, *do not* use that hair dye. This does not mean you cannot ever color your hair or use another color from the same manufacturer.

If you develop an allergic reaction to a particular dye, you are reacting to that exact molecular arrangement. There are so many possible variations in dyes that the next shade from the same manufacturer may be fine for you; but be careful: the same test has to be performed with every aniline dye you intend to use.

There are other do's and don't's that will ensure the best possible results from hair-coloring products:

SOME DO'S

1. Always wear gloves when you apply the dye to your hair. The hands can pick up the color of the dye.

2. Follow the coloring instructions of the manufacturer to the letter. Any deviation in procedure can easily cause poor results.

3. Apply the coloring agent to clean, dry hair unless otherwise directed by the manufacturer.

4. Always use a protein, acid-based conditioner after any coloring procedure. This will help to shrink the cuticle and restore the hair's elasticity.

5. If any dye gets into the eyes, wash out the eye area instantly, with plain warm water. If an irritation persists, consult your physician.

SOME DON'T'S

1. Don't massage the dye into the scalp; just work it through your hair. A hair-coloring agent is not a scalp treatment.

2. Never use a metallic or vegetable dye (often called color

restorers). The hair can become discolored or break off.

3. *Never* use an aniline dye on the eyebrows or eyelashes. Use only a product specifically designated for these areas, one that has no dye in it.

4. Never save an aniline dye mixture after it has been opened and/or combined with a developer. After coloring your hair, discard any remaining solution.

5. Don't have a permanent wave or straightening done on the same day as your hair coloring. Wait at least a week between each procedure.

How to Do Permanent Hair-coloring with Aniline Dyes

There are four basic methods for permanently coloring the hair that use aniline dyes:

1. Highlighting shampoo tints.
2. Shampoo-in tints.
3. One-step tints.
4. Two-step tints.

HIGHLIGHTING SHAMPOO TINTS: These are the easiest type of product to use. They are designed to cause a very, very slight change—just enough to highlight your own hair color. They are not suitable for covering gray hair. They contain a bit of peroxide, a shampoo, some oil, and an aniline dye.

Highlighting shampoo tints are applied to dry hair, worked through each strand, and left on the hair for a short time, usually five to ten minutes. Water is then added to make a lather, and the lather is worked through the hair like a shampoo. Finally, it is rinsed with warm water, and the hair is then shampooed once with a mild shampoo.

With this kind of permanent tint, the color is embedded in the cortex of the hair. The *highlights*, however, will change color and turn reddish because of the interaction of the air and the dye. To refresh the color, one should use a highlighting shampoo tint every five to six weeks.

Highlighting shampoo tints are good for people who want

to add a few highlights to their hair without changing its color. It is also an excellent treatment for very limp, straight, slippery hair that will not hold a set, because it contains enough peroxide to ruffle up the cuticle and give this hair more body. It will make this kind of hair look fuller, and the hair will hold the line of a set better. 5-MINUTE COLOR by Clairol is an example of such a product.

SHAMPOO-IN TINTS: These cause much more of a change than do the highlighting tints. They contain more peroxide, more dye, and a chemical "booster." This booster lightens hair and softens the cuticle, so that the dye can penetrate deeper into the cortex of each hair strand.

These tints also have a wider range of effects. One can pick a shade several tones lighter or darker than your own natural color. It is also possible to add a chemical called a *drabber*, which removes red highlights, a condition that plagues many women when they color their hair. Shampoo-in tint can be used to cover gray when there is no more than 30 percent gray hair on the head.

Shampoo-in hair color is applied to dry hair and worked into a lather through each strand. It is left on for twenty to thirty minutes, then water is added and the lather worked up again. It is rinsed out with warm water until the water runs clear. It should be followed by a mild, single-soaping shampoo, set, and dried.

To heighten the hair color without producing reddish highlights, a few drops of the drabber should be added to the hair-coloring mixture before it is applied to your hair; then proceed with your dyeing as usual. NICE AND EASY by Clairol and INNOCENT COLOR by Toni are both shampoo-in tints.

Shampoo-in tints make a permanent change in the hair color. But the original color of the tint will fade because of the continued effect of the air on the dye. After five or six weeks you may notice that the hair has lost some of its new highlights and color. At the same time the new hair growth around the scalp is coming up in your old color and the difference is noticeable.

Reapplication of shampoo-in tints follows the same procedure as the first application. There is no sectioning, as in one-step or two-step tints. The new color is applied all over the head. It covers the new growth and restores the lost color; it does not cause harsh buildup of color.

Shampoo-in tints are very easy and quick to use. They do not drastically change your hair, but after their use your hair looks brighter and the color seems deeper. It is especially useful for people whose hair color seems faded and dull. It is also good for brunettes, whose color looks drab. It can cover and blend in hair that is starting to turn gray. The application can easily be done at home and touchups are simple to perform.

ONE-STEP TINTS: With these, we start getting into professional-level hair coloring. These products are oil-based mixtures of peroxide, aniline dyes, and ammonia, and they lighten and color in one step.

One-step tints can effect a very noticeable change on the hair. For example, one can go from medium brown to bright red, from blond to blue-black, and from gray to golden blond. This kind of change is not possible with the products previously discussed. The choice of colors, however, is not totally unrestricted. One-step processing cannot make most hair colors convert to light-blond or pale-reddish shades. Within the range of one-step dyes, however, there are many effects that *can* be achieved.

One can choose colors with only gold highlights, only red highlights, or no highlights at all. Individual colors can be created by mixing different shades put out by the same manufacturer. However, this kind of shade selection should only be done by a professional hair colorist; it is a very delicate operation and takes years of practice and experience to do well.

Application of a one-step tint is a rather tricky proposition. Unless you are very skilled at working with your hands or have a friend who is, this should really be attempted only by a beautician. It is very easy to make a mess of it yourself.

First, the hair is divided into four sections on the scalp. Then the dye is applied to the hair, starting one inch away from the scalp. This is done because the heat of the scalp will make the hair near it color more rapidly. The dye remains on the hair for about fifteen minutes. It is then applied to the roots of the hair and the whole thing is left on thirty to forty-five more minutes.

Reapplication is also tricky. The hair is again divided into four sections. Dye is applied liberally to the root area, and left on for twenty minutes. A strand of hair is selected and the color observed. This is to see whether the new color on the roots comes out the same as the rest of the previously tinted hair.

The next step is to lightly comb the dye through your hair. The remaining dye in the bottle is then diluted half and half with a mild shampoo. This mixture is worked through the hair, and left on for just a minute or two. The final step consists of wringing this mixture out and shampooing with mild soap.

The one-step application lets you change your hair to almost any color except for the pale-blond and pale-red shades. It is the best choice for those who really want to change their hair color permanently, or who wish to cover gray completely.

Hair treated with the one-step process must be continually conditioned to prevent dryness and hair breakage. There are many strong alkaline chemicals used in this process and they must be counteracted with protein conditioners, acid-based shampoos and rinses, and warm-oil treatments. For further details, see the section "The Care of Artificially Colored Hair," pages 238–9. These hints will enable you to keep your hair soft, lustrous, and easy to manage after one-step tinting.

Examples of one-step tinting are MISS CLAIROL by Clairol and L'EXCELLENCE by L'Oréal.

TWO-STEP TINTS: This method has two distinct procedures: the first step bleaches out some to all of the existing pigment in the hair shafts; the second step adds dye or a toner to give the hair the final desired shade. This process is used almost exclusively for changing hair to the blond and light-red shades.

The hair is first treated with an ammonia and peroxide mixture, frequently called the lightener. This serves two purposes:

1. It lightens the natural hair color.

2. It makes the hair much more porous by swelling the hair shaft and raising the cuticle away from the rest of the hair shaft. This is necessary to let the dye, which is applied later, get into the cortex of the hair.

A lightener is left on from forty-five minutes to two hours. Even naturally blond hair must be treated for at least forty-five minutes to ensure sufficient swelling of the hair to permit entry of the dye.

When the first step is completed, the hair is rinsed, shampooed, and the toner is applied. The toner contains the dye that will give the hair its final color. When the hair is colored for the first time, a color-strand test should be made. The toning mixture should be applied to a single strand and left to develop for fifteen minutes. The strand is then rinsed, dried with a towel, and the color examined. This process should be repeated on the test strand until the desired shade has been reached. The length of time needed to achieve this color should be recorded and used to gauge how long the rest of the hair should be processed.

The hair is then sectioned, and the toner is applied with a small brush until the hair is completely saturated. The toner is left on the hair for the length of time determined by the strand test. The hair is rinsed out and conditioned, to finish off the procedure. The hair should be towel dried *gently*, and then set and dried.

With all the other hair-coloring procedures, the final shade was limited by the original shade of the hair. With two-step coloring, the original hair color is totally changed, so that theoretically a woman with jet-black hair can become a platinum blonde.

This transformation, however, can be far from desirable. From an esthetic point of view, the complexion and eye color of a dark-haired person might look sallow and unattractive with blond hair. From a practical point of view (the economic one), it may also be undesirable. Dark hair will need to be retouched at the roots very often, as often as once every ten days, if a pale-blond shade is to be maintained. Not only is this expensive and time consuming, but it can also be very bad for the hair.

Two-step processing is a very harsh treatment for the hair. It uses strong alkaline chemicals to swell, lighten, and color the hair. These damage the keratin of the hair and make the hair lose water. Frequent application at the roots (for example, every two weeks) will make the hair close to the scalp very dry and brittle. At this crucial point of stress the hair shaft can easily break off, and with considerable hair breaking off at the roots, the whole head of hair will soon look a lot thinner.

Processing will not stop or slow the normal rate of growth of your hair. But constant hair breakage can make it seem as though your hair is not growing as well as before. Even conscientious conditioning cannot completely prevent this kind of damage to hair that is heavily and frequently processed.

Two-step processing is good for those people who were

blond when they were younger. Their hair will be relatively easy to lighten, and they already possess the blonde's complexion and eye-coloring. In addition, the roots of their blondish-brown hair will not be as noticeable against the background of tinted hair, and reapplication is usually necessary only once every three to four weeks. The hair will therefore not be subjected to harsh chemicals as often, and will sustain much less damage. If you were a blond child and you wish to be blond again, two-step processing can give you beautiful, relatively easy-to-care-for blond hair.

Another group of people who can get wonderful results with this technique are the gray-haired women. Gray hair is really white hair mixed in with the original shade of hair color. The result to the eye is a grayish tone. Since the white hairs contain *no* pigment it is easier to lighten the hair.

Lighter hair shades are more becoming to the older face than dark browns or black, even if these were the original color. They provide a softer frame around the face, they make wrinkles less obvious, and they make the skin appear less sallow than do the darker hair shades. The gray roots do not contrast as harshly with blond hair. Dark-haired women who in their youth had wished to be blond can finally do so with a lot less bother than in their youth.

A second benefit of age is the fact that the hair begins to grow more slowly. This means that the roots will need touchup applications less frequently. Reapplication of dye can be stretched out to as much as once every six weeks without sacrificing the hair's appearance.

Frosting and Streaking

These are done in the same way as two-step processing; the lightening procedure followed by a toning procedure only on selected strands of hair is used. The color is removed from the strands and a toner applied to give it a blond shade. The final result is a mixture of hair color that gives brown or dark-blond hair a lighter appearance.

Lightening selected strands has many advantages. The major benefit is that there is no harsh line of demarcation of dark and light hair at the roots. Therefore, depending on the length of the hair, this procedure need be repeated only once every two to four months. Shorter hair, since it is being constantly recut, will grow out of its blond streaks much more rapidly than chin or longer length hair. The more time between applications, the less bother, expense, and damage to the hair.

Streaking and frosting are the best methods for brown-haired girls who were never blond to have blond hair. Streaking their hair gives the appearance of being lighter and brighter, without the problems associated with going *all* blond. In addition, the result is not as harsh a blond tone, and even if you have olive skin and dark eyes you can look quite attractive with this streaked effect.

Although the procedure is complicated, it is really not as difficult as the standard two-step dyeing, and it can be performed at home. There are special kits available just for frosting and streaking. If you do not like the results, the color will grow out without there being a line of demarcation at the roots. If you are not good at working with your hair, have it done at a salon.

Some colorists achieve an effect called a *sunburst*. This is a blending of different-colored streaks into the hair. The streaks are lightened as before. Some strands are tinted to different shades of blond, others to pale red, and still others to a darker brown. A mousy-brown head of hair can be turned into a lion-like mane of glowing blond-brown colors with this sunburst effect. The sunburst, however, is definitely not a do-it-yourself procedure.

Streaking and frosting do *not* give good results on gray hair.

Special Hair-coloring Problems

Most difficulties in hair coloring arise from the same central problem. It has been subjected to a series of permanents, strippings, dyes, and/or straightenings. It has many cracks in the cuticle. This kind of hair "picks up" too much color. The resulting color is splotchy and uneven. The hair is also brittle, dry, and dull.

This kind of hair must be reconditioned before it is tinted or waved. Any attempt to work with this type of hair before reconditioning will result in breakage, discoloration, and frizzing of the hair.

For details on reconditioning, see pages 238–40, the section on the care of artificially colored hair. There you will find formulas and programs to put life back into porous, tired hair.

There are special permanents for tinted hair and special dyes for permanent-waved hair usually available only in salons. If, at this moment, your hair—after many permanents, straightenings, or tintings—is brittle and dry, do not attempt to color or permanent it yourself. Use the conditioning treatments I suggest, but leave all other procedures to experienced hairdressers. They have the products and the techniques that will normalize your hair and allow it to take on coloring in a healthy way.

If your hair is in good condition you can color and permanent-wave it at home, but never do the two at the same time. Always wait a week between each procedure.

The Care of Artificially Colored Hair

Most hair bleaches and coloring preparations contain very alkaline chemicals that cause little cuts on the surface of each hair.

Look at the drawing below. Diagram 28A is of unprocessed hair. Notice that the cuticle (the outermost layer) is smooth and even. The hair looks shiny to the naked eye. But now look at B. Notice how rough and ragged the hair's surface is. This is because the alkaline bleaching or coloring solutions have literally taken pieces out of the individual hairs, leaving the surface of each hair strand rough and flaky.

Why does this make your hair look dull? Imagine a still, shining pond. You can see your reflection in it because, on such a smooth surface, the light rays are reflected evenly enough to form

Diagram 28.

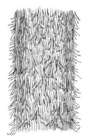

A. UNPROCESSED HAIR

The surface of unprocessed hair is flat, smooth, and shiny.

B. PROCESSED HAIR

The surface of processed hair is ragged and dull.

a mirror image. When you throw a pebble into the pond, the surface becomes rough and you can no longer see yourself; this is because the light rays are no longer able to form a mirror image.

The same thing has happened to bleached hair. When its surface is rough and flaky, the light is not reflected evenly, which causes the hair to look dull.

Special Problems of Bleached Hair

Constant bleaching also makes the hair dry and brittle. Bear in mind that hair is very much like the top layer of the skin. In order to remain smooth and flexible, the skin needs water. So does hair.

The water molecules in the hair keep it stretchable and soft. The chemical changes resulting from the bleaching remove water from the hair. The hair becomes stiff and weak. These water-poor hairs break off easily, split at their ends, and feel brittle to the touch.

A common way of handling such hair is to use hair oils and pomades. As with the skin, the oil acts as a shield against evaporation. And, in addition, the hair oil fills in the cracks and makes the cuticle seem less flaky and irregular.

But oil is only a temporary camouflage. To bring back the natural bounce and sheen to bleached hair, one needs to know more about what causes bleached-hair problems.

Dyed or tinted hair has lost the ability to maintain the proper water level. When the hair is wet, the cracks in the hair cuticles let it absorb too much water. The hair becomes sodden, heavy, and is just as prone to breaking off as when it was dry. Just feeding water to the hair will not make it well. At the same time, the highly alkaline bleaching process lifts the cuticle away from the rest of the hair strand. This produces a loosely formed hair fiber that lets the hair lose too much water while drying, just as it allows the hair to take in too much water while wet.

Bleaching damage must be attacked on several fronts:

1. The alkaline effects of bleaching must be neutralized with acidic shampoos.

2. The cracks in the cuticle must be filled in with a protein conditioner.

3. The water level must be helped with sauna-oil treatments. An acid shampoo will tighten up the hair strand and make it stronger. It will also enable the hair to maintain a good level of water in its shaft. Proteins in a shampoo provide a layer of amino acids on the hair and fill in the cracks where alkaline substances have destroyed the hair protein.

This is not to say that protein shampoos can "regenerate" the hair shaft. Hair has an affinity for proteins similar to its own natural proteins, and properly formulated protein shampoo will be taken up by the hair and will make it stronger and shinier. These proteins act like a varnish on the hair strand. They coat the hair and make it better able to regulate its water supply. They give it a smoother surface which will reflect light evenly. The effect is cumulative, and after several months a good, firm layer of these proteins is built up on the hair, making it healthy, flexible, and shiny.

The hot-oil treatment (see pages 250–1) is very useful as a gentle, gradual means for getting water back into each strand. The oil contains a great deal of dissolved water. When you heat the oil slightly and apply it to the hair, and then wrap the head in a hot wet towel, you are in effect creating a mild sauna. This heat releases the water molecules from the oil, and this water penetrates into your hair. The oil coats the hair so that the water cannot evaporate from the individual strands.

A PROGRAM OF CARE FOR BLEACHED HAIR

ONCE A WEEK

1. Wash with an acid shampoo, such as AMINO-PON shampoo by Redken.

2. Rinse off, and apply for a second shampooing.

3. Work up a lather, and rinse.

4. Apply a protein or balsam conditioner.

5. Leave on for twenty minutes.

6. Rinse with lukewarm water.

7. Add more conditioner, and again let it remain on your hair for twenty minutes.

8. Rinse out.

. . .

Special Problems of Dyed Hair

DANDRUFF: Dyed hair is as likely to develop dandruff as any other type of hair. The standard sulfur-based anti-dandruff shampoos, which are the most effective, can further damage hair that has already been weakened by bleaching. The best kind of dandruff shampoo for weakened hair contains zinc pyrothione. This is found in HEAD & SHOULDERS by Lever Brothers and in BRECK ONE by Breck. These are excellent products for dandruff but are unfortunately alkaline, so that if you use one of them it is wise to follow it with an acid shampoo or conditioner.

A DANDRUFF TREATMENT FOR DYED HAIR

1. Wet hair.

2. Apply one of the zinc pyrothione-containing shampoos.

3. Rub the shampoo into the scalp—do not try to cover hair, but concentrate on the scalp.

4. Leave on for three minutes.

5. Rinse off well.

6. Apply acid shampoo.

7. Rub into your hair and let it sit for three minutes.

8. Rinse out well.

9. Apply protein and/or acid-based conditioner.

10. Set your hair.

THE SUN: Dyed hair is easily damaged by the sun. The sun's dehydrating heat and ability to break up keratin fibers can make a mess of otherwise well-conditioned hair.

Protection can be obtained in several ways. The best way is total coverage. Always wear a towel wrapped around your hair, or a large hat on your head, when out in the sun. Be sure to wear a bathing cap while swimming.

A second way to protect your hair is simply to rub into the hair a good sunscreen lotion that you would normally use on your face or body. A good product of this type is PRESUN by Westwood Pharmaceuticals. It should be washed out as soon as you get out of the sun. A good treatment for sun-damaged hair is on pages 219–20.

PERMANENTS: Dyed hair is very often hard to permanent-wave, especially when it is dry and brittle. The hair must be brought back into proper condition before any attempt can be made to wave it. A special crash program should be initiated for at least six weeks before waving. The hair should be shampooed and treated with protein-containing, acidic products. Once each week, follow this program:

A "CRASH" PROGRAM OF CARE FOR DYED HAIR YOU WANT TO WAVE

1. Brush your hair, starting with the back of the neck. Give your scalp a finger massage or use a vibrator.

2. Wet your hair with lukewarm water. Do *not* use hot water. This will make your damaged hair even more fragile.

3. Pour on your protein shampoo.

4. Work the shampoo into your hair and scalp.

5. Rub the scalp so that it moves.

6. Rinse out your hair in a basin of water. Do not let a blast of water from the shower take off the shampoo. The force of the water can break fragile hair.

7. Pour water over your head.

8. Pour two ounces of condensed milk on your hair.

9. Mix one ounce of protein or balsam conditioner with one tablespoonful of oil.

10. Pour this mixture over the milk on your hair, wrap head with clear plastic wrap.

11. After one hour, rinse out with cool water.

12. Set.

Go through this routine once a week for at least six weeks before attempting to permanent your hair.

IMPORTANT DON'T'S FOR DYED HAIR

1. *Do not use a cream rinse on dyed or tinted hair.* These contain a small amount of quaternary ammonium salts, which can weaken the dyed hair. These ingredients are used

to soften the hair enough to separate tangles and make it easier to pull a comb through your hair. It is too strong a product for dyed hair.

Use protein conditioners, preferably those that are acidified, but avoid anything that promises mainly to "soften hair" or "remove tangles."

2. *Do not use products based on herbs.* The natural dyes in these plants can discolor dyed hair.

Permanent-waving

Permanent-waving, or cold-waving, is to the hair what plastic surgery is to the face. It can give body to limp hair, make thin hair seem thicker, and give waves and curls to straight hair.

Carefully done and carefully conditioned, chemically waved hair can look beautiful and healthy while holding its style or line much better than it could before. Badly done, the same process can cause considerable damage to the hair. It can make the hair so dry and brittle that it breaks off. Hair in this condition is dull, very difficult to set, and almost impossible to tint properly.

How a Permanent Wave Works

Remember that the protein molecules of the hair are held together by chemical bonds or links. The way these bonds position the protein molecules, which make up the building blocks of the hair shaft, determines the straightness or curliness of the hair. For example, with very straight hair, the protein molecules and the chemical bonds are parallel to each other, while with curly hair the bonds and protein molecules are at right angles to each other (see Diagram 26, page 182).

If you want to change straight hair to curly hair, you must rearrange the position of the protein molecules and the bonds that connect them. You must break the bonds and reset them so they are at the desired angle to the protein molecules that they connect.

There are three basic steps to hair waving:

1. Wrapping the hair in a small roller.
2. Breaking the protein bonds.

3. Re-forming the protein bonds at new angles.

Wrapping your hair in rollers stretches it slightly, and makes it more vulnerable to having its bonds broken. The wrapping of your hair around a small round roller gives it a new curved pattern when the protein bonds begin to re-form.

The breaking of bonds is accomplished by the use of a waving lotion. This is a highly alkaline solution that contains *ammonium thioglycolate*, the compound that actually does the bond breaking. Lanolin and proteins are often included to condition the hair. The alkalinity of the waving lotion softens the hair shaft and makes it easier for the ammonium thioglycolate to enter the shaft and disrupt the bonds.

The roller-wrapped hair is totally saturated with the waving solution. The time necessary for the bonds to break varies with the condition of the hair, the strength of the waving lotion, and the type of wave desired; it ranges from four minutes to half an hour.

When the right amount of time (determined by the kind of hair you have—see pages 245-7) has passed, the hair, still wrapped in rollers, is rinsed with water. Excess waving lotion is blotted off with a towel, and a *neutralizer* is applied.

A neutralizer is composed of peroxide and lanolin. It stops the chemical action of the waving lotion, and encourages re-formation of chemical bonds in their new positions. Because it is acidic in nature, it encourages the hair shaft to become firm and strong. After several minutes of being neutralized, the hair is removed from the rollers and shampooed.

Formerly straight hair will now have waves when wet. Set and dried, this new wave pattern will allow the hair to hold a set much longer than before the permanent-wave.

The size of the rollers and the strength of the waving solution used in the permanenting determine the size of the finished wave. The larger the roller and the weaker the solution, the larger and softer the waves will be.

A cold-wave using the largest possible rollers and the weakest available solution will give a very soft result called the *body wave*. This procedure causes just the smallest change in the positions of the protein molecules and their chemical bonds. It is used for people who wear their hair smooth and straight but who desire a longer-lasting set.

A mild body wave can make very thin hair seem much

thicker. The strongly alkaline waving solution swells the hair shaft and raises the cells that form the cuticle. This increases the diameter of the hair shafts. If each hair is thicker, then the whole head of hair will also seem thicker and fuller.

Hair Characteristics to Consider for Waving

To get the best results from a permanent, five basic characteristics of your hair must be analyzed: hair porosity, thickness of the hair shaft, hair elasticity, hair volume, and hair length.

HAIR POROSITY: This is the ability of the hair to absorb fluid. It is a major factor determining the length of time a waving solution should be left on your hair. The quicker the hair takes up the liquid, the more porous it is, and the less time is needed for the waving solution to be absorbed into the hair.

Porosity is determined by the tightness of the cuticle, the outermost layer of the hair shaft.

With virgin hair—that is, hair of a young person that has never been waved or colored—the cuticle is very tight and smooth. The hair in this condition is not very porous, and it will take a longer period of time for the waving solution to be absorbed.

As one grows older, even if the hair remains untreated, the cuticle becomes less smooth or even. Little cracks and chips form on the surface of the cuticle, making these hairs more porous than virgin hair. This kind of hair has what is called average porosity; it gives the least trouble during the waving process.

Hair that has been frequently lightened, tinted, or waved is very porous. It quickly absorbs the waving solution and great care must be taken to prevent overwaving—which results in frizzy, dry, stiff hair. A very mild lotion left on the hair for a very short time is the only kind of waving this kind of hair should receive.

Hair that has been heavily lightened and had too frequent wavings, and is, as a result, dry and brittle, is overporous hair. No attempt should be made to wave this hair. A concentrated program of conditioning treatments carried out over several months can restore some of the health to this damaged hair. It can then be waved with a very mild solution. Any attempt to wave this hair without conditioning can result in baldness.

THICKNESS OF THE HAIR SHAFT: The diameter of each hair will also play a part in determining how quickly the waving solution will be absorbed. Very thin hair, having a smaller shaft diameter, will absorb the waving solution more rapidly than thick hair. However, a thick hair that is porous will absorb fluids more rapidly than a thin hair that is not as porous. When it comes to a choice between the two, the porosity is a more important factor to consider than the thickness of the hair.

HAIR ELASTICITY: Elasticity is the natural capacity of the hair to stretch out and contract. The water content of the hair determines its stretchability as well as its flexibility. When adequate amounts of water are present, the hair is flexible, it takes a curl well, and to the touch it seems soft and bouncy.

When there is loss of water, as after waving, coloring, or exposure to the sun, the hair becomes stiff and brittle. At this point the hair has lost its elasticity. Such hair is very difficult to wave. It refuses to hold a curl.

HAIR VOLUME: The more hair there is on the head, the larger the rollers must be to give a good wave, and, of course, there will have to be a large number of them. If insufficient rollers are used, the hair will not be stretched and patterned properly, and a poor wave will result.

Thin hair—that is, hair that is reduced in numbers—needs smaller rollers than does average hair. And, like very thick hair, it needs many rollers, but for a different reason: Too many hairs from a sparsely populated scalp attached to a single roller can cause excessive strain on the hair.

HAIR LENGTH: The techniques outlined for waving hair are appropriate for hair no longer than six inches. When hair is more than six inches long, special problems arise.

Longer hair, hair that reaches down below shoulder length, must be wound several times around a single roller. This results in a great deal of tension on the hairs that are closest to the roller, while the outer hairs, those that are farthest from the roller, will experience very little pull at all. At the same time, with a great deal of hair wound around each roller, it is very hard for the waving lotion to reach down and act on all the hairs wrapped on the roller.

Under the circumstances, it is almost impossible to obtain a firm curl wave. However, long hair will take a soft, body-type wave, which gives the hair better curl retention and more body.

To achieve the desired wave, the above five different hair characteristics must be weighed against one another. Only then can one decide what the strength of the waving solution should be and how long the solution should remain on the hair.

This is a fairly complex balancing process, since it involves a good deal of judgment and experience to attribute the proper value to each of these characteristics. It takes a skilled hairdresser to tell what sort of waving lotion will be best for your hair.

Hair-waving Mistakes

Home waving kits rarely give as good a result. Many cases of overwaving or underwaving have resulted from the use of these preparations.

The manufacturer is not at fault, since the products themselves are perfectly adequate. Most people, however, lack the technical skills needed to use them properly. For example, it is very hard to put the rollers on evenly over the back of your head and it is very important that each roller be equally saturated with the same amount of lotion. One has to work very quickly in order to apply the lotion evenly and at the same time to the entire head, so that each strand of hair is treated for the same length of time. If it takes too long to put the lotion on, the front of your head will be more processed than the back.

The end results of a clumsy application are overprocessing or underprocessing. Of the two, underprocessing is less of a problem. Underprocessing is simply a sign that the waving lotion has not done its job; the hair has only very shallow and weak waves. The hair is not damaged, but neither is it waved.

This hair should be treated with a conditioner and the waving process tried again in a few days. Better care in the saturation of the rollers and the timing of the wave solution will produce a good wave pattern. Underprocessing rarely occurs in a beauty salon, and is usually the result of a do-it-yourself job. Any attempt to rewave should always be done by a hairdresser. Be sure to mention the earlier unsuccessful attempt to the hairdresser, who will adjust his or her approach to your hair.

Overprocessing is just about the worst thing that can happen to your hair besides losing it. The hair has the appearance, texture, and shine of a used steel wool pad. It is dry, stiff, frizzy, dull, and brittle. It can break off easily, making the hair seem thin and sparse.

This sad state results from improper treatment with the waving lotion. Too much lotion was used, it was too strong a solution, it was left on for too long a time, or it was not properly neutralized. The alkaline nature of the waving lotion has damaged the protein molecules themselves, and the hair has become weak and fragile.

Overprocessed hair is terribly curly when wet, and frizzy and matted when dry. This damage cannot be reversed. The hair can be reconditioned with protein rinses and shampoos; these will restore some of the shine and elasticity, but the hair will remain very curly. The only solution is to wait for the hair to grow out and cut off the permanented ends.

Overproceessing can, of course, occur in a beauty parlor with an inexperienced hairdresser, but it is much more likely to occur when the permanent is done at home.

How Often Should a Permanent Be Done?

Short hair that is frequently cut to maintain its style will grow out most of the permanented hair in two or three months. It will need a new permanent wave every three months to maintain a firm curl.

Longer hair, which is not cut as frequently, needs a wave every six months to supply body and curl. A very soft body wave should also be repeated every six months.

Six months is the maximum time that the effects of any permanent wave can be noticed. After that, so much new hair has grown, or old waved hair has been cut off, that the hair conforms pretty much to its old shape.

The Care of Permanented Hair

A soft body-type wave puts very little strain on healthy hair, so it is not necessary to follow any special conditioning program. Follow the normal system of care depending on your type of hair (e.g., dry, oily, normal). However, a curly wave, the result of longer contact with the waving lotion, does need conditioning.

The chemicals used in waving are strongly alkaline. They attack the keratin of the hair itself, thereby causing many cracks in the cuticle, which makes the hair appear dull (because it loses its mirror-smooth surface). In addition, these chemicals draw water out of the hair, leaving it desperate for moisture. Without moisture, the hair loses its stretch and flexibility. It becomes stiff and brittle. It has a great tendency to break off. When this happens, the remaining hairs look sparse and thin on the scalp.

The best way to prevent this disaster is to condition permanented hair after each shampoo. This means using acidic hair products to keep the cuticle smooth and tight. At the same time, protein shampoos and conditioners should be applied frequently in an attempt to strengthen the hair shaft. Finally, hot-oil treatments using moisturizing lotions should be undertaken once a month (see pages 250–1).

A PROGRAM OF SHAMPOOING AND CONDITIONING FOR PERMANENTED HAIR

1. Brush hair, but not as thoroughly as with unprocessed hair.

2. Use an electric scalp vibrator to stimulate blood circulation in the scalp, a job that deep brushing would ordinarily do.

3. Use only acid shampoos, even if your hair is oily.

4. Rinse all the soap out of your hair.

5. Blot gently.

6. Apply a conditioner. Be very fussy about the one you choose. Do not use a cream rinse: it contains chemicals that soften the hair, and the last thing permanented hair needs is something that softens the hair fiber. The hair is soft and weak enough already. Do not use a conditioner that is

mainly a body builder or hair-setting lotion. Nor should you use one that is really a hairdressing cream. A hairdressing cream, which is rubbed into the hair after it is dried and set, results in crisp, frizzy, but nonetheless oily hair.

Look for a conditioner that is creamy, but liquid, that is applied to wet hair and is specifically designed for bleached or waved hair. Two such products are Redken's P.P.T. 77, and Clairol's CONDITION. These products will feed water and water-hungry substances to the parched hair and provide a coating to discourage evaporation of water. Conditioners of this type also close the cracks in the hair's cuticle, making the hair shinier and smoother.

5. After conditioning, set your hair. No setting lotion is necessary.

6. Dry hair under a hair dryer set at medium heat, not hot.

7. When dry, remove clips and rollers and brush out and set. The hair can now be styled.

8. Use a light dusting of hair spray. This is not so much to hold the line of coiffure as it is to encourage the hair to hold moisture. The hair spray coats the hair with a plastic coating that slows down the evaporation of the hair's moisture.

Once a month give yourself a special conditioning treatment—the *hot-oil treatment*, described below. In this process a warmed, water-rich lotion is applied to the hair and a hot towel is wrapped around the head. After twenty minutes, the towel is removed and the oil is washed out of the hair. There are several products specially designed for this treatment, but a thin, all-purpose lotion, like NIVEA or LUBRIDERM can be used just as successfully and much less expensively.

THE HOT-OIL TREATMENT

1. Heat one fourth of a cup of the lotion (more if your hair is long) over a double boiler until it feels hot to the touch. *Caution*: Do not allow it to boil or even simmer—that would be much too warm and could actually burn your scalp.

2. Apply this preparation to your dry hair, with a clean paintbrush.

3. When the hair is well saturated with cream, wrap a large hot towel around the head, turban style. In order to make the towel hot, soak it in very warm water and wring it out. Cover towel with aluminum foil to keep heat in.

4. After ten minutes, replace the towel with a fresh hot one, and keep it on the head for another ten minutes.

5. Rinse with lukewarm water and wash with a mild shampoo.

6. Set and dry.

This treatment will keep permanented hair healthy. But if, right now, your hair is dry, frizzy, thin, and unmanageable, dull, lifeless, and faded, you need more help.

The Care of Hair Damaged by Permanent-waving

A crash program of moisturizers and protein body builders is needed for weak hair. After each weekly shampooing (this hair should not be washed more often) a concentrated protein treatment should be applied. Such protein conditioners are usually thick, expensive, and packed in single-application treatment units. They are meant to be left on the hair for between fifteen and thirty minutes before being rinsed out. One such product is EXTREME PROTEIN PACK by Redken. It is very expensive, at about two dollars a treatment, but it does contain proteins that coat the hair shaft, thereby filling in the cracks made by the waving solutions. With these cracks filled in, the water stays in the hair, and the hair thus becomes softer and shinier.

At the same time, this coating, by increasing the diameter of each hair, makes the whole head look fuller and thicker, a bonus for those people with thinned hair as a result of permanent-wave damage. The coating strengthens the hair and decreases the possibility of breakage.

. . .

A SPECIAL PROTEIN TREATMENT FOR HAIR DAMAGED BY PERMANENT-WAVING

1. Shampoo the hair with one sudsing. Rinse.
2. Apply the protein conditioner directly to the hair.
3. Let it remain on for thirty minutes.
4. Rinse out with tepid water.
5. Shampoo again.
6. Set and dry.

Once a month give yourself the hot-cream treatment described previously.

Damaged hair needs additional special care. It must *always* be shielded from the sun by a hat or scarf. The sun can cause additional protein damage and dehydration, both of which are very harmful to hair damaged by permanent-waving. When your hair is in poor condition, no further waving or coloring should be done until a series of reconditioning treatments has restored its elasticity and strength. This can be difficult going if your hair has been colored, and a ban on tinting can lead to an ugly showing of roots. The only thing I can suggest is to wear a wig when the line of root demarcation becomes too visible. Additional processing can lead to disaster. All the hair can break off, leaving you bald or nearly so.

After the hair begins to look and feel better (usually after two to three months) you can touch up the hair colors; but do not use a bleaching and toning process. Instead, use the simple one-step coloring procedure to even out the hair color. Do not permanent this hair even now. Wait until all the permanented hair has completely grown out, and new, healthy hair has replaced it. When your hair has been fully restored, follow the preventative conditioning program (pages 249–51) to avoid the "dull, dry brittles."

Hair Straightening

Hair straightening is a process whereby curly, frizzy hair is made straighter and smoother. It is based on the same principles as hair waving and uses the same chemicals—the strongly alkaline ammonium thioglycolate waving lotion, and an acidic neutralizer.

The waving lotion breaks the existing curly pattern of molecules in the hair. The hair is then subjected to the pull of gravity and hangs straight. The waving lotion is called the *relaxing lotion* in the hair-straightening process, because that is exactly what it does—it relaxes the tight, curly structure of the hair so that it uncurls and hangs straight.

The neutralizer locks the hair molecules in this new form, making new bonds, and the whole straightening process is completed.

A TYPICAL HAIR-STRAIGHTENING PROCEDURE

1. The hair is washed out with a neutral shampoo, towel dried until the hair is slightly damp, and then combed free of tangles.

2. The thick, creamy straightening lotion is applied with the hands protected by rubber gloves.

3. The straightening lotion is spread all over the hair, great care being taken not to rub it into the scalp. It is a very caustic solution that can burn and blister the scalp, as well as the skin of your face or hands.

4. It is left on the hair for about twenty minutes, the exact length of time depending on the texture and the curliness of your hair.

5. The bonds of the hair are now broken. Now is the time to reshape the hair. With hair waving, you will recall that this restructuring is done by having the hair wound around rollers while the lotion is applied, thus re-forming the hair in a curved position. By contrast, with hair straightening the object is to rearrange the hair in a *straight* position. To this effect, after the relaxing lotion has remained on for about twenty minutes, the hair is combed straight for ten to twenty minutes. A comb is slowly and continuously run through the hair, encouraging it to hang straight.

6. A neutralizer is now smoothed on with the gloved hands, taking care to maintain the hair in a straight, untangled state. This is now also combed through the hair for several minutes. The neutralizer fixes the hair in its new straight shape, and strengthens the hair after its harsh bout with the straightening chemicals.

7. The straightening lotion is rinsed out of the hair. Make sure the hair remains straight and smooth on the head.

8. The hair is then set on giant rollers and dried under a hair dryer.

Hair Characteristics to Consider for Straightening

To get the best possible results from a straightening, four basic characteristics of the hair should be analyzed: hair porosity, thickness of the hair shaft, hair volume, and hair length.

HAIR POROSITY: This is the ability of the hair to absorb fluid, and is a major factor in determining the length of time a relaxing lotion should be left on your hair. The quicker the hair takes up the liquid, the more porous it is and the less time is needed for the relaxing solution to be absorbed into the hair.

Porosity is determined by the tightness and lack of cracks in the cuticle, the outermost layer of the hair shaft.

With virgin hair—that is, hair of a young person that has never been straightened or colored—the cuticle is very tight and smooth. Virgin hair is not very porous, and it will take a longer period of time for the relaxing solution to be absorbed.

As one ages, even if the hair remains untreated, the cuticle becomes less smooth and even. Little cracks and chips form on the surface of the cuticle and make these hairs more porous than virgin hair. Such hair has average porosity, and gives the least trouble during the straightening process. There is less danger that the hair will not straighten or absorb too much relaxer and become damaged.

Hair that has been previously lightened, tinted, straightened, or exposed to a great deal of sun is very porous. It quickly absorbs the relaxing lotion, and great care must be taken to prevent an overabsorption of the lotion, which leads to stiff, extremely brittle hair that readily breaks off. This breakage can cause a very noticeable decrease in the volume of hair on your head, and it will make the hair seem sparse and thin. With such hair, the straightening lotion is left on for the shortest period of time possible. It is better to settle for slightly wavy hair rather than to try for board-straight hair and then wind up with no hair at all.

Hair that has been heavily treated with bleach and/or too frequent wavings and is thus dry and brittle is overporous. No attempt should be made to straighten this hair. A concentrated program of conditioning treatments carried out over several months can restore some of the health to this damaged hair; then, and only then, can the hair be straightened with a very mild solution. Any attempt to straighten this hair without conditioning can easily result in extensive loss of hair.

THICKNESS OF THE HAIR SHAFT: The diameter of each hair also plays a part in determining how quickly the relaxing solution will be absorbed. Very thin hair with a smaller shaft will absorb the relaxing solution more rapidly than thick hair. However, a thick hair that is porous will absorb fluids more rapidly than a thin hair that is not porous. When it comes to a choice between the two, porosity is more important to consider than the thickness of the hair.

HAIR VOLUME: The more hair there is on the head, the more lotion and the longer the time necessary to achieve good results. The hair has to be thoroughly saturated with the solution. The amount of lotion correct for thin hair will be inadequate to straighten a fuller head of hair. Thick hair needs a longer combing time to be successfully treated than does thin hair.

HAIR LENGTH: Hair longer than eight inches presents two problems. It obviously requires more relaxing lotion; it is also much more difficult to keep straight and untangled during the application of lotions, combing, and rinsing. It also takes a longer time to comb the relaxing lotion through long hair.

To achieve the proper straightening and good health of the hair, these four characteristics must be weighed against one another. A decision involves a good deal of keen professional judgment and experience, and this is an excellent reason for not attempting do-it-yourself straightening at home.

While many of the principles of hair waving are identical to those of straightening, the latter process creates problems uniquely its own.

As mentioned earlier, the straightening solution is very

caustic and will often irritate the scalp. This irritation can be minimized by first applying cold cream or solidified mineral oil around the hair line, which generally is the site of the worst irritation.

Another problem with the straightening lotion concerns the length of time it has to remain on the hair. The total time varies from a minimum of twenty minutes to over an hour, quite a bit longer than the time necessary for cold-waving, which at the very most is thirty minutes. This long time is needed because the straightening demands that the majority of the bonds in the hair be broken. The lotion remaining on the hair for such a long time can cause severe damage. In fact, the straightening process is probably the roughest thing you can do to your hair. It is much more damaging than bleaching, waving, or even stripping the hair of color during a bleach treatment.

Because of the danger, special precautions and care must be taken with straightening. It is inadvisable to use any coloring but a semi-permanent tint on straightened hair. The permanent dyes are too strong, too alkaline for such hair. Since the semi-permanent dyes do not contain peroxide or ammonia, they do not affect the protein of the hair as does a permanent dye.

Straightened hair must be vigorously protected from sunburn, chlorine pools, and salt water. And sulfur dandruff shampoos are too strong for this kind of hair. The milder but still effective zinc pyrothione shampoos (e.g., BRECK ONE) should be used instead.

Home hair straightening is far too difficult and delicate to be done even by a gifted amateur. Salon straightening is usually a little more expensive than permanent-waving, but it is cheaper in the long run, since it is done much less frequently. Total straightening should never be done more often than once every six months. Touchups around the hair line, where the new growth of curly hair appears, can be done every four months. When the hair has been touched up, however, total restraightening should be done only once yearly.

The care of straightened hair is much the same as that of permanent-waved hair. The straightening lotion weakens the protein structure of the hair and causes cracks in the cuticle, the outermost layer of the hair, which makes for dull, dry hair. The cracks in the cuticle also allow water to evaporate from the hair. Without water the hair loses flexibility and bounce, and becomes stiff and brittle.

Care of straightened hair entails the strengthening of the hair structure as well as a shrinking of the hair shaft back to normal in order to make it less susceptible to losing water. Acid shampoos will shrink the hair shaft back to normal, firm up the protein, and fill in some of the cracks.

A PROGRAM OF CARE FOR STRAIGHTENED HAIR

1. Shampoo according to the instructions on page 181. Brush your hair thoroughly, as with unprocessed hair. Use only acid shampoos, such as AMINO-PON K-11 by Redken.

2. Rinse all the soap out of the hair.

3. Blot gently.

4. Apply a conditioner, but be very careful about your choice. Do not use a cream rinse, because it contains chemicals that soften the hair, and the last thing straightened hair needs is a softened hair fiber. In addition, you cannot use a conditioner that is mainly a body builder or a setting lotion. Nor should a cream hairdressing be used. This is the type of oily conditioner that is rubbed into the hair after it has been set and dried. Straightened hair has a tendency to hang limply —and a greasy cream will only make it limper.

Look for a protein conditioner that is creamy but liquid when applied to wet hair, and specifically designed for bleached or waved hair. Three such products are Redken's P.P.T. 77, Clairol's CONDITION, and Mennen's PROTEIN 21. These conditioners will feed water, and water-hungry substances, to the thirsty hair and provide a coating to discourage evaporation of water. Conditioners of this type also close the cracks in the hair's cuticle, making the hair shinier and smoother.

Straightened hair has a tendency to become brittle. But instead of becoming bushy and "flyaway," straightened hair often hangs limply. A hot-oil treatment that is food for dry brittle hair would only make straightened hair limper. The brittle, fragile quality of straightened hair is helped by a special protein treatment like Redken's EXTREME PROTEIN PACK. This kind of conditioner will coat each strand with a film of protein, giving added support to weak hair.

Glossary of Cosmetic Ingredients and Terminology

Alcohol: Alcohol is found in soaps, deodorants, skin fresheners, and acne products. It has strong grease-cutting (dissolving) properties and is a good disinfectant.

Women with *dry* skin should assiduously avoid cosmetics containing alcohol.

Astringents containing alcohol are frequently prescribed as part of a regimen for acne care, primarily because of their grease-dissolving properties. However, the bacteria involved in acne problems are found deep in the pores and are not affected by the topical (surface) application of alcohol. Be on the lookout for acne-care products that contain only alcohol. They cannot do nearly as good a job as a preparation containing, in addition to alcohol, sulfur, resorcinol, and/or salicylic acid.

Alcohol when present is listed on the label.

Allantoin: Allantoin is a chemical extracted from the comfrey root. It is an anti-irritant, with healing and soothing properties, which is used in diaper-rash creams, moisturizing lotions, and sunburn preparations.

It has no antiseptic properties.

It is not considered a major cause of cosmetic allergies and is frequently a valuable additive in face creams, masks, and lotions. Its presence must be noted on the label of any product in which it appears.

Almond Oil: This is a vegetable oil extracted from bitter almond seeds. It stays fresher longer than many other similar nut oils, and is, for this reason, used in many commercial products.

It does not commonly cause allergic reactions.

This product must be distinguished from the fragrant extract of oil of almond. The latter product is used primarily as a perfume and is a cause of allergic reactions.

Alopecia: This term refers to the absence of hair from skin areas where it is normally present.

Althea: This is an herb said to have emollient properties. It can be used in a dilute infusion for sunburn and for dry skin.

Infusion: A brew of herbs. To one cup of boiling water add one tablespoonful of herb. Let this mixture steep for twenty minutes. Strain and cool for one hour. Apply the preparation with a cotton pad to the dry or sunburned areas of the skin.

Alum: This is an aluminum salt widely used in facial astringents, mouthwashes, and aftershave lotions.

It is the chemical in an astringent that gives it its pore-reducing abilities. It acts by creating a slight swelling of the skin. The puffed-up skin rises and surrounds the pore, obstructing it from view. After several hours, the edema subsides and the pore is then visible once again.

The presence of alum is very important to the efficiency of an astringent. Unfortunately, the F.D.A. does not require this ingredient to be listed on a cosmetic label. You can write to a manufacturer for a list of the ingredients in his astringents. If he refuses to give you such information, you can add ½ teaspoon of powdered alum (available from a supermarket) to eight ounces of the astringent you already have.

Aluminum Sulfate: A common aluminum salt, used in astringents and mouthwashes. Very similar to alum. Sometimes the two words are used interchangeably. See *Alum* for more information.

Amino Acids: These are the chemical building blocks of protein that make up many of the fundamental parts of our body, including the skin and the hair. The formation of skin from amino acids (and other basic building materials) is an extremely complex process. Rebuilding the skin through the application of creams containing amino acids is strictly for science fiction; there is no way the skin can utilize these chemicals to produce new skin.

Shampoos and hair conditioners containing amino acids are another story. The surface of the hair accepts these broken-down parts of protein and uses them to fill in the cracks in the hair shaft caused by alkaline soaps and harsh processing. These new proteins do not rebuild the hair shaft; they simply add support, like plaster to a cracked wall.

Ammoniated Mercury: This is a bleaching agent that acts to reduce skin color by preventing the formation of melanin. It is not a very effective way of dealing with skin discoloration and, in addition, has several potential bad effects on the skin. Many allergic reactions have been ascribed to this chemical.

It is now banned in cosmetics by the F.D.A.

Ammonium Thioglycolate (thio = relaxer): A chemical hair relaxer that breaks the chemical bonds of the proteins giving your hair its shape. Used in products designed for hair waving and hair straightening.

Aniline Dyes: These chemicals are derivatives of coal tar and are used primarily in hair dyes. In sensitive persons these products have been known to cause blindness when used in the areas around the eyes.

These dyes are found in almost all permanent hair-coloring products. One must always do a patch test each time such a dye is used. The presence of these dyes in a product must be listed on the label.

Anise: An herb said to have soothing properties.

Antiseptic: A chemical agent that prevents the growth of bacteria. Examples of antiseptic chemicals are alcohol, iodine, and hexachlorophene.

Apples: Fresh apples and fresh apple juice contain vitamin C, and an enzyme, amylase, that can peel the skin to some degree.

Just what, if any, properties apple extracts in a commercial cosmetic product retain is unknown. In all probability, both the enzyme and the vitamin content of the fresh fruit are destroyed and the acidity overwhelmed by the alkaline components of the cosmetic preparations containing the so-called fresh apple extracts. All that's left in these products is an apple fragrance. Any product that claims to contain apple extract owes whatever value it has to its other ingredients.

Arcels (see also *Spans, Tweens):* These are substances used as emulsifiers in creams, lotions, and sunscreens. They keep the oil molecules and the water molecules together, maintaining a nonseparating product. They have no effect on the skin itself. They are meant to refine the product physically, not to improve its action on the skin.

Arnica Flowers (also known as *Leopard's Bane, Wolf's Bane,* or *Mountain Tobacco):* Arnica consists of the dried flower of a plant found in northern Europe, Asia, and North America. It has been used for the local treatment of bruises and sprains, and sometimes as an astringent.

Arnica can be fatal if taken internally, and can cause allergic reactions in many people. It should not be used in cosmetics. There are many other safer substances that are good astringents and that do not have the bad side-effects of the arnica flowers.

Artichoke: The artichoke appears in cosmetics primarily as an oil. As such, it is an average vegetable oil and has no special properties other than the basic emollient properties of any vegetable oil; it is not as useful an emollient as an animal oil. Personally, I would much rather have my artichoke hot with lots of hollandaise sauce. In this way it will do a lot more for my spirit than it could possibly do for my skin.

Astringents: These are cosmetics specifically designed to make the pores of the skin *seem* smaller. The most important ingredient in such a product is an *aluminum salt*. This chemical causes a mild swelling of the skin, which results in the temporary disappearance of a pore.

Astringents also contain water, preservatives, perfume, and coloring. Other commonly included additives are alcohol, camphor, witch hazel, glycerin, salicylic acid, zinc salts, herbs, and mint extract, all of which add distinctive properties to the basic astringent (see individual listings for the purpose of each additive). (See also recipes for dry-skin astringent, pages 40 and 44; oily-skin astringent, pages 49–50; acne astringent, page 59.)

Attar of Roses: An extract of roses used to perfume a product. This additive has been known to provoke allergic reactions.

Avocado Oil: A vegetable oil with no special properties, either when fresh and applied directly to the face or as a preserved extract in a commercial product. This oil in no way warrants the current cult that has been created as a result of the promotion campaign alluding to its special benefits.

The avocado itself is, however, especially delicious in a green salad into which you have added crumbled bacon and chopped red onion.

Azulene: This is a substance extracted from camomile flowers. It has soothing properties and is found in face, hand, and body creams, suntan remedies, burn ointments, bath salts, and cosmetics designed to be nonirritating. Its presence is valuable as an anti-inflammatory agent, to soothe irritated skin. It has dubious value, however, as part of a product that is supposed to prevent irritation due to the product itself. The skin will become irritated because of the presence of irritants. Azulene in the same product will not prevent such a reaction.

B21: The advertised ingredient in one of the most expensive creams on the market ($85 for 2½ ounces at the last check). According to the manufacturer, B21 is actually a code name for a mixture of vitamins. The 21 does not represent any one vitamin (there is no vitamin B_{21}) nor does it mean there are 21 vitamins in this product. The 21 was selected, according to the manufacturer, in honor of the company's twenty-first anniversary.

Balm Mint: This additive, though sometimes found in cosmetics, is not mentioned in any of the major references in the cosmetic chemistry literature.

Balsam of Peru: See *Peru Balsam.*

Bananas: Bananas have been put into creams, soaps, and face masks. The extract of banana is quite worthless for the care of the skin. Banana oil is a typical vegetable oil. It can form a film on the face that cuts down water evaporation from the surface of the skin but it has no special properties. Freshly mashed bananas is the best preparation for the use of this oil, but is messy to use. All in all, bananas are much better eaten than smeared on the face. I am quite partial to banana fritters that are laced with cognac.

Beeswax: This compound is a secretion of the honey bee and is extracted from the honeycomb. It is widely used in cosmetics as an emulsifying agent—that is to say, it permits the solid and liquid chemicals in a beauty product to combine in the form of a homogeneous substance (as in a smooth cream or lotion). Without an emulsifier, the cosmetic would quickly separate, leaving the solids at the bottom and the liquid ingredients on top.

Benzoic Acid: Benzoic acid is used as a preservative. It is not considered irritating to the skin, although it may cause an allergic reaction in persons sensitive to similar chemicals.

Bergamot Oil: This oil is extracted from the rind of citrus fruits. It is used in the manufacture of eau-de-cologne and other perfumes. It is also used as a fragrant additive in creams and lotions. Unfortunately, the combination of bergamot oil and sunlight causes a skin rash in a significant number of people.

Biodynes: See *Biostimulants.*

Biostimulants (also called Filatov extracts): These are substances extracted from the tissues of plants or animals that have been subjected to stressful situations, such as extreme heat or cold. It is felt that under such circumstances an organism reacts by producing a substance that helps its cells to survive. This substance is promoted as being very beneficial in the "rejuvenation" of aged or wrinkled skin, but there is great controversy as to the actual value of these extracts. The exact secretion that these cells under stress are supposed to produce has never been isolated. People who work with biostimulants simply mush up the "stressed" cells and extract a mixture of many substances, one of which is believed to be "biostimuline." It is virtually impossible to gauge the amount and/or strength of the substance present. There are many conflicting reports as to its effectiveness. Even more controversial is its power to renew old skin. However, protein extracts from animal cells have been reported to cause severe allergic reactions. It is wisest to stay away from biostimulants until much more research on them has been done.

Biotin (vitamin H) or *Biotine:* A deficiency of this vitamin has been associated with greasy scalp and baldness in rats and other experimental animals. However, fur-bearing animals (such as the rat) have a very different hair growth than human beings. Biotin deficiency in man is extremely rare.

It is considered a worthless additive in cosmetic products.

Birch: An herb whose value, if any, to skin and hair has yet to be determined.

Bluing Rinse: A solution used to neutralize the yellowish tinge that accompanies gray hair. (See recipe, page 214.)

Body Builders (for Hair): These are usually weak solutions of hair spray. The sticky resins in the hair spray coat each individual hair shaft, giving these hairs extra width. Body builders with protein work on the same principle. The proteins attach themselves to the *outside* of the hair shaft, giving it extra width. The hair often has a special affinity for protein and is more likely to hold on to a coat of protein for a longer period of time than to a hair-spray-based body builder.

Borax: This is a white, odorless mineral. It has mild cleansing properties and is slightly antiseptic. It is most often used as an emulsifier in cold cream. It is also used in mouthwashes, vanishing creams, bath salts, eye lotions, cleansing lotions, and scalp lotions. It has not been shown to cause allergies.

Boric Acid: It is prepared from sulfuric acid and natural borax. It has fair-to-good antiseptic properties and has been used in talcum powder. In the past it has been widely used as a dressing for wounds and burns. Some deaths have resulted from too great an absorption of boric acid in patients with extensive wounds or burns, and it is no longer a favorite antiseptic in the treatment of these problems. It has also been removed from baby products.

Butyl Stearate: This is one of the most common stearic acids used in cosmetic formulation. It is used in nail polish removers, lipsticks, and cleansing creams.

It has been shown to be a cause of allergic reactions.

Cactus (also *Irish Moss*): This plant possesses two distinct properties. It has a sticky, gelatinous quality that is very valuable in a face mask. Most of the clear peel-off masks contain this kind of substance. In addition, it is also a good emulsifier; for this reason it is used in the manufacture of some creams and lotions.

Cactus does *not* have any special health-giving properties. It cannot change or correct the biology or chemistry of your skin.

Calamine Lotion: This solution of minerals has mildly astringent and cooling qualities. It is particularly useful for sunburned or irritated skin.

Camomile: This is one of the very few herbs that have any real value for the hair or skin. A mild infusion of camomile leaves produces an oily substance that is soothing to the skin. A concentrated solution of camomile left on the hair for one to two hours will lighten the hair by several shades.

Camphor: This product is obtained from certain tropical trees that grow primarily in Java, Sumatra, Japan, and Brazil. Camphor is quickly absorbed by the skin and produces a feeling of warmth followed by a mild sensation of numbness.

Camphor is useful as an antiseptic, it soothes itchy skin, and is, moreover, a rubefactant (it reddens the skin).

Camphor is used for chapped skin and as a counter-irritant in liniment rubs, where it warms and soothes sore muscles.

Canities: This is the medical term for whiteness or grayness of the hair.

Capsicum: A red pepper that when processed for use on the skin exerts an irritating effect on the skin. It is used in hair tonics to stimulate hair growth and as a counter-irritant in muscle rubs.

Carbolic Acid: An extremely caustic acid that is sometimes used in chemical face peeling. It may lead to severe scarring of the face.

Carbolic Soap: This is a disinfectant soap containing about 10 percent phenol. It is used for the management of oily skin.

Carnauba Wax: This wax is extracted from the pores of the leaf of the carnauba palm tree, which grows in Brazil. It is used to firm up substances such as cosmetics, giving them a less fluid consistency. It is found in creams, depilatory waxes, and deodorant sticks. It does not usually cause allergic reactions.

Carrot Oil: Rich in vitamins, this oil has essentially the same properties as any other vegetable oil.

Casein: This is a protein derived from whole milk. Casein is used in cosmetics as an emulsifier, particularly in massage creams. The skin does not absorb casein and it does not exert any effect on the health of the skin.

Castile Soap: This soap uses olive oil as its primary source of fat. It has no unique properties and can be used successfully by people with normal or slightly dry skin.

Castor Oil: This is a vegetable oil extracted from the seeds of the *Ricinis communis* plant. It has the same properties as other vegetable oils. Because of its unpleasant odor, it is not widely used in cosmetics. However, because it is rarely, if ever, associated with irritation of the skin or allergic reactions, it has some use in medical-grade creams or pastes as well as in several types of eyedrops.

Certified Color: This is a dye the government guarantees safe in any quantity used. Recent investigation of these certified colors, however, tends to indicate that they may not be as harmless as claimed. The F.D.A. is reviewing the list and some of these colors may be dropped from the list.

Cherry Laurel: This is an herb thought to have soothing properties on the skin.

Chlorophyll: This chemical is found in the cells of green plants. It has been said to be useful as an aid to the healing of wounds. It is widely used in toothpastes, mouthwashes, and deodorants to protect against odors.

Cinnamon: It is said to have a soothing effect on the skin.

Citric Acid: This chemical is present in citrus fruits. It is used in bleach creams, hair rinses, bath salts, bubbling denture powders, and in a few astringents. Citric acid is not usually irritating to normal skin, but it can cause burning and redness when applied to chapped, cracked, or otherwise inflamed skin.

Citronella: This substance is derived from the fragrant grass *Cymbopogon nardus* of Asia. It is used both as an insect repellent and in perfumes. Some cases of skin sensitivity have occurred with this chemical.

Clay: This mineral is used in face powders, body powders, face masks, and foundation for makeup. It does not cause skin allergies. It is good for oily, acne-troubled, and normal skin.

Clover Blossom: This herb is said to have astringent qualities.

Cocoa Butter: This oil is extracted from the roasted cocoa nut seeds. It has the same emollient properties as any other vegetable oil. Cocoa oil has been associated with allergic reactions.

Coconut Oil: This oil is frequently used in soaps because it produces a good lather. Skin irritation occurs in some people when they use this oil.

Cod-liver Oil: This animal oil contains vitamins A and D. Some healing and antiseptic properties have been attributed to the presence of the vitamins, but the use of this oil in cosmetics is limited because of its unpleasant fishy smell.

Corn Oil: A vegetable oil with average emollient properties. Corn oil does not seem to excite the imagination of cosmetic companies, and magic claims have not been inflicted on this oil. Corn oil is a good inexpensive oil that is not particularly prone to cause allergies.

Cornflower: This is an herb said to have astringent properties.

Cucumber: Cucumber extracts contain vitamin C and chlorophyll, and are naturally acid. However, although fresh cucumber may be beneficial in some cosmetics, the usual commercial extract is so heavily processed that it no longer contains any of its initially beneficial ingredients. Fresh peeled cucumbers are, however, delicious with yogurt and a pinch of cumin.

Developers: These are oxidizing agents (usually containing hydrogen peroxide) that supply oxygen to the molecules of a hair-dye solution, allowing the dye to achieve a particular color.

Eggs: The presence of eggs in a cosmetic is purely a promotional gimmick. The skin cannot utilize the protein contained in an egg.

A fresh egg mask creates a watertight film on the face and allows the skin to build up a good supply of water. This water will temporarily soften dry skin. (See "Dry-skin Mask I," page 44.)

Elder: This is an herb said to have astringent properties.

Embryo Serum: This rather nightmarish substance is extracted from the chopped-up bodies of unborn chicks. It is used in wrinkle creams, face masks, and special injections that are supposed to remove lines and wrinkles.

These embryos, as the theory goes, contain "youthful" hormones that can rejuvenate the skin. This is nonsense. Nothing rejuvenates the skin. The tiny amounts of hormone usually present in commercial face creams and masks probably have no effect on the skin whatsoever. The proteins derived from the embryo, on the other hand, may cause severe allergic reactions and even death.

Estrogen: This is a female hormone produced by the ovaries. It is used in night creams, which are promoted for dry and lined skin. In low doses, which are permitted by the F.D.A., estrogen does not alter the *growth* of skin cells. It does, however, encourage the skin to hold on to extra water, and is therefore a useful ingredient in a cream used on aging lined skin.

Medical-grade estrogen creams contain several times the amount of estrogen allowed in over-the-counter cosmetic creams. There is some evidence that in this dosage estrogen does improve skin tone to a limited degree.

Eye Cream: Almost every line of cosmetic offers a special night cream for the eyes. This is a useless product, since the undereye area does not have unique problems that call for a different kind of night cream from that used for the rest of the face.

Fatty Acids: These are a group of chemicals that are extracted from fats such as wheat germ oil, sunflower seed oil, sesame seed oil, poppyseed oil, and corn oil. Sometimes cosmetic companies call fatty acids vitamin F. This is quite incorrect, since fatty acids are not at all like vitamins.

There is no evidence to prove or, for that matter, to believe that fatty acids have special value to the skin or hair. In fact, fatty acids have been shown to be the real culprit in acne problems. Anyone with oily skin or acne should make a special effort to keep away from cosmetics that contain fatty acids.

Fennel: This herb is thought to act as a mild antiseptic.

Fenugreek: This herb is thought to have emollient properties.

Filatov Extracts: See *Biostimulants.*

Filler: This is a preparation used to recondition processed hair before retreatment.

Ginseng: This is the dried root of *Panax schinseng.* It is reported to contain vitamins, hormones, and some special growth substance. The Chinese believe it to be an aphrodisiac.

There is no evidence that ginseng can improve the appearance of the skin. It has, however, been associated with many allergic reactions of the skin.

Glutamic Acid: There is an extremely expensive cosmetic that claims its special powers come from the fact that it contains both glutamic acid and an amino acid that in combination are supposed to do wonderful things for your skin. Just to set the record straight, glutamic acid *is* an amino acid. Amino acids, which are the building blocks of proteins, only combine to form protein under certain chemical conditions, and more than two amino acids are needed to form just about any protein useful to the body. Therefore, simply having glutamic acid and/or any other amino acid present in a night cream is worthless. The whole idea, so vigorously promoted by the cosmetic advertisers, that you can rebuild the proteins of your skin with amino acids is pure malarky.

Glycerin: This is a clear, syrupy liquid made by chemically combining water and fat. The water splits the fat into smaller components, glycerol and fatty acids.

It is used in many cosmetics and toiletries. It improves the spreading qualities of creams and lotions and prevents them from losing water through evaporation. Glycerin has a tendency to draw water out of the skin and can make dry skin drier. It has not been shown to cause allergies.

Grapefruit: Fresh grapefruit juice contains vitamin C and is very acidic. As such it is too caustic to use on the skin and face. Commercial products that advertise grapefruit in their contents usually extract an essence or oil from the rind of grapefruits. This part of the fruit contains no vitamin C but does contain fertilizer and insecticide residues. These may provoke acne in certain sensitive people.

Grapes: These contain vitamin C, chlorophyll, and enzymes. Despite this "impressive" array of natural ingredients, however, the grape extract that finds its way into cosmetics has been so reprocessed that it is useless. It is far better to drink the "grape" than to spread it on the face or hair.

Green Soap: Green soap is made of potash, glycerin, and olive or linseed oil. It has strong grease-dissolving properties and is good for oily skins.

Hand Creams: These contain alcohol, stearic acid, lanolin, and gum substances.

They are basically vanishing creams with extra oils added. They do not need to be as greaseless as those used under makeup.

Hard-water Soaps: These contain coconut oil, borax, sodium silicate, and a phosphate. These soaps are very alkaline. They are designed to lather and clean in areas where the water contains a great deal of un-dissolved minerals.

Hazelnut: This is an herb said to have astringent properties when applied to the skin.

Henna: This is made from the powdered leaves of the Lawson plant before the plant sprouts flowers. It is used primarily to impart reddish highlights to the hair. It has not been shown to cause allergies on the scalp but can do direct damage to the hair. A full discussion of henna is found on page 227.

Honey: Honey is composed primarily of sugar and wax. It has no special properties for the skin. However, masks that contain honey create a watertight film on the face and permit the skin to rehydrate itself.

Hormo-fruit Extracts: These are extracts from germinating plants, which supposedly contain growth hormones. There is no evidence that plants indeed do contain such substances.

Horsetail: There is no evidence that this herb has any effect on the skin or hair.

Hydrogen Peroxide: A colorless liquid that can potentially "burn" the skin. It is used primarily in hair dyes, where it has a two-fold action. The hydrogen peroxide breaks down the melanin in the hair shaft, making the hair a lighter color. It also releases oxygen, which combines with the small aniline dye molecules and helps them develop their color.

Irish Moss: See *Cactus.*

Juniper: An infusion of juniper is said to have rubefactant properties.

Lanolin: This is an oil extracted from the wool of sheep. It is inexpen-sive and is used in many cosmetics.

      Lanolin is one of the best oils for use in cosmetics. Its composition is closest to that of sebum, which is the oil secreted by the human oil glands. It provides excellent protection against water evaporation from the skin and hair but does not interfere with any other cellular processes.

      Raw lanolin has been shown to cause allergies in some people. There is a special process that makes lanolin less allergic, and this is the kind of lanolin used most frequently.

Lavender: Lavender is said to have healing properties.

Lecithin: This substance is used primarily as an emulsifier. It has no special dermatologic activity even though it is found in the skin. There is no known condition caused by lack of lecithin.

Lemon: Lemon contains citric acid and vitamin C. It has good degreasing abilities. It is one of the few living substances that can retain its properties after chemical extraction. One must be careful that a lemon cosmetic contains concentrated lemon juice and not just essence for a lemony smell.

Freshly squeezed, strained lemon juice mixed with water is an excellent rinse for oily hair. (See recipe, page 189.)

Lettuce: It is said to have emollient properties in its fresh state, but after processing for use in cosmetics it is unlikely to retain this property.

Linden: Is said to have soothing properties when applied to the skin.

Mallow: This is an herb said to have soothing properties. It is used in shampoos and a few creams.

Malt (also *Hops, Beer):* Malt has rubefactant properties in a cosmetic because of the presence of yeast. It is used in face masks and toning lotions.

Massage Cream: This is frequently a plain cold cream with a little extra soap added to make it less oily and a bit stickier—to give the masseur a better "grip."

Melissa: An herb said to have soothing properties.

Milk: There is absolutely no evidence to indicate that milk in a cosmetic has any effect on the skin. The skin cannot absorb or utilize the protein contained in milk. Milk in cosmetics has no effect on the growth of skin, the formation of lines and wrinkles, or the skin color.

Casein, a protein found in milk, is used as an emulsifier in the manufacture of cosmetics.

Milk is used in permanent-wave neutralizers to reduce irritation to the scalp. This is probably the only active role that milk plays in any beauty product.

Mineral Oil: This is a clear, odorless oil derived from petroleum. It is the most widely used oil in cosmetic formulations. Mineral oil is inexpensive and never causes allergic reactions.

Mint: This is an aromatic herb widely used as a fragrance in beauty products. Spirit of mint, an alcohol extract of mint, has rubefactant properties and is used in face masks and toning lotions. In some cases spirit of mint has been shown to be irritating to the skin.

Mistletoe: There is no mention of mistletoe in medical literature and it is doubtful that it is of any cosmetic aid.

Moisturizer: Moisturizers generally contain water, mineral oil, lanolin, emulsifiers, and sometimes water-holding substances. Moisturizers provide a source of water for the skin and a protective layer of oil that shields the skin against the evaporation of water. They do not contain as much soapy emulsifier as do thicker creams.

Nasturtium: A flower said to have rubefactant properties.

Natural Cosmetic: By dictionary definition, a natural product must contain one or more substances that were originally living things. In cosmetic terminology the term "natural" usually means anything the manufacturer wishes. There are no legal boundaries about the term, and a manufacturer may call any product natural. Usually a natural cosmetic contains a vegetable oil, or plant extracts. Occasionally, "natural cosmetics" might use vitamin E as a preservative. As a whole, natural cosmetics are purely an advertising gimmick.

Nettle: This is a plant rich in vitamin A. It has been used in face creams and shampoos.

Nonalkaline Soaps: Soaps that have an alkaline pH (defined as a pH greater than 7) dissolve protein as well as keratin. People with dry skin have very flaky keratin. Alkaline soaps are thus very bad for dry skin.

     Some nonalkaline soaps include:

     1. Dove (Lever Brothers) is superfatted and contains detergent and pH = 7.

     2. Lowilla (Westwood), pH = 4.

     3. pHisoderm (Winthrop) contains detergent, petroleum, lanolin, and cholesterol, pH = 5.5.

     4. Aveeno Soap substitute (Aveeno), pH = 6. 65 percent Aveeno colloidal oatmeal and petroleum are the major ingredients. There is no soap or detergent.

     5. Soy Dome Soapless Cleanser (Dome), 10 percent soya flour, with detergent, pH = 5.

Nucleic Acids: These are found in the chromosomes of the body. They are very specific chemicals that act only in the nucleus of cells. There is absolutely no way a solution of nucleic acids applied to the skin's surface or to the hair can have any effect on their appearance. Any claims to that effect are fraudulent and should be reported to the F.D.A. or the F.T.C.

Nutrient Cream: This is a product supposed to "feed" the skin and make it healthier. The skin, however, cannot "eat." All the skin's nutrients must be absorbed from the blood stream.

Oatmeal: This grain contains a colloid that has soothing properties on the skin. Oatmeal-based preparations are given by dermatologists for irritated skins resulting from, say, sunburn, psoriasis, or allergic dermatitis. The oatmeal seems both to subdue the irritation and to relieve itching.

Oatmeal is also used in face masks and soaps. Oatmeal masks absorb oil from the skin's surface and reduce the redness of irritated, broken-out skin. Oatmeal soaps are nonirritating and are good for people with sensitive skin. There are oatmeal soaps advertised for acned skins, but these are not nearly as good for this skin problem as are soaps containing salicylic acid, resorcinol, or sulfur.

Olive Oil: This is a vegetable oil with no special properties. It is used in the manufacture of castile soap.

Orange Flower: This flower is said to have soothing properties.

Organic: By dictionary definition, an organic substance is a living plant or animal that has not been grown with feedings of hormones or other chemicals, and has not been exposed to pesticides. In cosmetic terminology, organic means whatever the manufacturer wishes. Sometimes an organic cosmetic contains plants, vegetables, fruits, or herbs; in other instances, organic means the product does not contain preservatives; and frequently the term organic is nothing more than an advertising come-on.

Ozone Gas: Many cosmetologists have a machine that sprays the skin with ozone gas. Ozone will kill some of the bacteria on the skin's surface. This can be done just as efficiently, however, by rubbing alcohol on the surface of the skin. Furthermore, the alcohol found in a strong anti-acne soap can do the same job at a much lower cost. Ozone cannot rejuvenate skin, diminish lines or wrinkles, stimulate circulation, or any other such marvelous claim. And, in fact, there is evidence that prolonged exposure to even small amounts of ozone may be harmful.

Pantothenic Acid: This is one of the B vitamins. It is found in liver, eggs, dried brewer's yeast, and the royal jelly of bees.

Pantothenic acid does not pass through the skin's barrier. Its main claim to fame is the belief that it can prevent gray hair. This idea was based on some experiments with rats, but these results do not apply to human hair, probably because rats and humans have very different hair growth cycles.

There is no evidence that pantothenic acid in cosmetics has any effect on the skin or hair.

Papaya: Papaya contains the enzyme papain, which has the ability to dissolve keratin. Papain is used in face masks and peeling lotions, which are designed to remove the top layer of skin. It is frequently the active ingredient in "exfoliating lotions" and "vegetal peels."

Papain can be irritating to the skin, but is less so than bromelin, a similar enzyme found in pineapples that is also used in cosmetics.

Parsley: Is said to have disinfectant properties.

Peptides: A combination of two or more amino acids. Peptides have no value in skin preparations but are useful in shampoos and conditioners. The peptides in these products form a film on the individual hair shafts, making the hair seem thicker; in addition, by their coating action they help to retain moisture, they fill in cracks in the hair shaft, and they strengthen it and make it shinier.

Peptones: A protein formed in the body during digestion. An example of a peptone is casein, derived from milk (see casein for its use in cosmetics).

Peptones in general have no value when applied to the surface of the skin or hair.

Peru Balsam: This is a sticky liquid extracted from the bark of a South American tree. It has two very different applications in beauty products:

1. It is a strong rubefactant and is used in hair tonics to stimulate the circulation of the scalp.

2. Balsam also has the ability to form a clear, hard film when it dries. This property is at work when Peru Balsam is used in shampoos, cream rinses, and conditioners. The balsam forms a thin shield on the outside of the hair strand, gives support, and helps the hair maintain a good supply of water.

Petitgrain: Is said to have soothing properties.

Petroleum Jelly: This substance is used in products meant for chapped, raw skin. It is an inexpensive substance that provides an excellent shield against water evaporation. It is very mild and has not been shown to cause allergies or irritation.

Phenol: Phenol is a derivative of carbolic acid. It is an extremely caustic chemical and is considered undesirable for use in cosmetics. Even at low concentrations phenol frequently causes irritation.

Phenol frequently is used for chemical face peeling, the dangers and benefits of which are discussed on pages 85–7.

Pine: Acts as a rubefactant when applied to the skin. It can be irritating and cause red splotches.

Pineapple: Contains bromelin, an enzyme that dissolves keratin. It is used on the face in masks and peeling lotions to remove the top layers of the skin.

Placenta Extract: Placenta extracts contain many vitamins and female hormones that have, under certain circumstances, been shown to help the appearance of the aging skin. But, and it is a very big but, there is the question of how much vitamin or specific hormone is present in a given placenta cream. The F.D.A. requires the listing of the concentration of vitamins and hormones in any such product. I have yet to see a cosmetic containing placenta that lists these components.

The placenta itself does not contain the essence of youth just because it is associated with birth. The value of a cosmetic depends on its ingredients (hormones, vitamins, etc.) and it is impossible to tell if you are getting your money's worth. You are much better off buying a vitamin cream or an estrogen cream; you will know exactly what you are getting.

Plantain: A banana-like fruit that is said to have astringent properties.

Potatoes: There is no commonly accepted evidence that potatoes have any external value for the skin or hair.

Progestin: A derivative of progesterone (a female hormone). In creams this hormone encourages the skin to hold onto its moisture.

Raspberries: The essence of these sweet, refreshingly scented red berries is added to cosmetics to give them the fruit's fresh smell. Sometimes these products claim to have therapeutic value for the skin because of the presence of raspberries. There is no evidence that raspberries can have any external value for the skin. In fact, raspberries are fairly allergenic as fruits go, and their presence in a product can increase its allergenicity. Fantastic with sugar and *crème fraîche.*

Resorcinol: This is a chemical substance of great value in skin care. In very mild solutions, it is used as an antiseptic and as a soothing preparation for itchy skin; in slightly higher concentrations, it removes the dry dead layer of the skin's surface.

Resorcinol is used in lotions for irritated skin and particularly in connection with acne. While it is a very good ingredient for the care of skin, it can cause irritation in some people. And it may alter hair color in blonds.

Robane: This is a "hydrogenated squalene," which means that it is a saturated fat similar to cholesterol. It has the same properties as animal fats, and thus is one of the more desirable fats. It is frequently used in night creams.

Rose Hips: This extract of roses is rich in vitamin C. For its value see *Vitamin C.*

Rosemary: This herb is said to have rubefactant properties.

Roses: The extract of this flower is said to have astringent properties. Essence of roses is frequently used as a fragrance in toiletries.

Royal Jelly: This substance is found in beehives. It is secreted from the digestive tube of worker bees. The male bees and the workers eat royal jelly for only a few days after they are born, but the queen bee eats royal jelly all of her life. Because royal jelly is associated with the health and long life of the queen bee, it was believed that this substance could have some age-retarding properties.

It does not—there has been extensive research on the value of royal jelly and the scientific consensus is that it is worthless for humans Anyone who claims that it has special powers is a fraud.

Sage: This herb is said to have healing properties.

Salicylic Acid: This is a chemical found in some plants, particularly the leaves of wintergreen and the bark of sweet birch. It is an extremely useful additive in many cosmetics. It is an antiseptic, and dissolves the dry dead layer of cells on the skin's surface. It is widely used in acne soaps and lotions as well as in dandruff shampoos.

Sandalwood: There is no evidence that sandalwood has a beneficial effect on skin or hair.

Sea Water: There is no evidence that any of the components of sea water have any special value for the skin or the hair.

Seaweed: This plant has gelatinous properties. It is the major ingredient in the thin, clear masks that peel off in one piece. The mask allows the skin to build up a supply of water.

Seaweed is also used in face creams and lotions, where it gives body and substance to the products.

Sesame Oil: This oil has the same emollient properties as other nut or vegetable oils. Sesame oil, however, blocks 30 percent of the burning uv rays of the sun, and is extremely useful in suntan lotion. Plain sesame oil offers better protection than many more expensive suntan-preventing products.

Shark Oil: An animal oil with large quantities of vitamins **A** and **D**. This oil has good emollient properties (as do all animal fats), but its use is restricted in cosmetics because of its fishy odor. Products that contain shark oil usually have only very small amounts of this oil because of the smell; the only value of these cosmetics must come from their other ingredients.

Silicones: These are minerals with the ability to repel water. Silicones are used in toothpastes, where they form a water-repellent film on the teeth that prevents staining by food or tobacco.

Silicones are used in face creams, where they increase the products' protection against water evaporation from the skin. Silicones are also used in shampoos, where they are felt to help the hair maintain better water balance.

Silicones are not irritating, they are inexpensive, and they are in general a good ingredient to look for.

Soaps: See *Nonalkaline Soaps; Superfatted Soaps.*

Sodium Lauryl Sulfate: A detergent used both as a cleanser and as an emulsifier in creams and lotions. Some people are allergic to it.

Sorbo: An emulsifying chemical used in the manufacture of cosmetics.

Spans: Emulsifying chemicals used in the manufacture of cosmetics.

Speedwell: There is no evidence that this herb is of any cosmetic value.

Spermaceti: This is a waxy substance obtained from the head of the sperm whale. It is used in the manufacture of cosmetics, to thicken the products and give them shine. It is nonirritating.

Stimulines: See *Biostimulants.*

Sulfur: This is a mineral that is extremely valuable in skin and hair care. It has the ability to slow down oil-gland activity, and to dissolve the top layer of dry dead cells. For this reason it is widely used in acne soaps and lotions as well as in dandruff shampoos. While it is the major ingredient in many acne and dandruff preparations, it can cause allergic skin reactions and hair breakage in some sensitive people. It is not the same as *"sulfa,"* an abbreviated form for a group of antibacterial agents, including sulfadiazole, sulfathiazole, etc. The two are sometimes confused.

Superfatted Soaps: These types of soaps contain additional fat or oil for the specific purpose of preventing excessive defatting of dry skin. Such soaps are probably less drying than ordinary ones because their detergent properties are less marked. The better a detergent, the more defatting it is; consequently, adding a fat to a detergent makes it a less effective cleanser, and more oil remains on the skin.

Examples of superfatted soaps include:
1. Basis (Duke)—2 percent lanolin.
2. Oilatum Soap (Stiefel)—7.5 percent peanut oil.
3. Superfatted Soap (Stiefel)—6 percent lanolin.

Swan Oil: Swan oil is supposedly what keeps swans afloat. Since swans can no longer be killed for sport or profit, synthetic swan oil has been developed. The synthetic oil is made up animal and vegetable oils and is probably no better than any other combination oil product. It does not have additional properties to justify its high price.

Tannic Acid: This chemical is present in tea. It has a healing effect in minor burns, and is also a mild astringent. Tannic acid is used commercially in burn ointments and sunburn remedies.

Thymol: This is a derivative of phenol and is antiseptic. It is used in the care of psoriasis, eczema, and acne.

Tomatoes: There is no evidence in the medical literature that the application to the skin or hair of tomato or its derivative compounds has any value.

Turtle Oil: This oil is extracted from the genitals and muscles of the giant sea turtle. Turtle oil contains very small amounts of vitamins. It has no special value for the skin other than the film-forming properties common to all oils. Turtle oil is one of the oldest cosmetic gimmicks. It was discredited as early as 1934, but somehow cosmetic companies are still putting out this oil complete with great promises. It is really time that the turtle oil hoax be put to rest.

Tweens: Emulsifying agents used in the manufacture of cosmetics.

Vitamin A: This is probably the most important vitamin to the appearance of the hair and skin. Vitamin A can pass through the skin's layers and may exert an effect on the rate of keratinization of the skin and hair. Vitamin A is a valuable additive in acne preparations, dry skin care, dandruff shampoos, and in soothing creams for burns and irritated skin. While it is important to have enough vitamin A, very serious problems can result from too much vitamin A. When using vitamin A, be sure not to exceed the minimum daily requirements in the total amount you take by pill or apply to your skin.

Vitamin B$_1$: This vitamin cannot pass through the layers of the skin and is of no value in skin or hair care preparations.

Vitamins B₂ and B₆: These vitamins also do not penetrate the skin and have no value in cosmetic preparations.

Vitamin C: There is some evidence (contested by other doctors) that this vitamin can pass through the layers of the skin and promote healing of tissue damaged by burns or injury. It is found in burn ointments and creams used for abrasions.

Vitamin D: This vitamin is absorbed through the skin's outer layers. There is some evidence demonstrating that vitamin D exerts a healing effect on the skin when applied topically. It seems to work particularly well when it is combined with vitamin A. Vitamin D is used in diaper rash remedies and in burn ointments.

Vitamin E: This seems to be the vitamin fad of the year. Whatever value or lack of value vitamin E has when taken internally, it has absolutely no value when applied to the skin's surface or to the hair. Vitamin E does not penetrate the skin's outer layers. All its claims for healing powers are without true scientific foundation. In fact, there is evidence to show that when vitamin E is forced through the layers of the skin (as with spray-on preparations) it can cause severe allergic reactions. The F.D.A. is considering a total ban on vitamin E from cosmetics and toiletries.

Vitamin H: See *Biotin.*

Vitamin K: This vitamin does not pass through the skin's outermost layer and is of no value in skin or hair preparations.

Watermelon: There is no evidence in the literature to indicate that watermelon is of any value to the skin or hair.

Wheat Germ: This grain is used in cosmetics because of its large content of vitamin E. See *Vitamin E.*

Wild Ginger: There is no evidence to indicate that this herb has any value in beauty care.

Witch Hazel: This consists of the dried leaves of the shrub *Hamamelis virginiana.* The active ingredient in witch hazel is *tannin,* whose properties were discussed under *Tannic Acid.* However, the clear commercially distilled extract of witch hazel, which is widely available, contains only minute quantities of tannin. Any properties this extract may have come from its high concentration of alcohol. The witch hazel in it only provides the pungent odor.

      The alcohol extract of witch hazel is a red-brown liquid containing large amounts of tannin. This extract has an astringent and soothing quality. Extract of witch hazel is also found in hemorrhoid creams and in liniments.

Yarrow: There is no evidence to indicate that this herb has any effect on the skin or the hair.

Yeast: See also *Malt.* Yeast has a rubefactant effect on the skin. It is used in face masks designed to give the skin a ruddy color. It is good for pale, sallow complexions, but can be irritating to dry or sensitive skins.

Ylang: Ylang is an herb said to have emollient properties.

Yogurt: There is no evidence that yogurt applied to the surface of the skin has any lasting beneficial effect. It does have rubefactant properties and can be used in a homemade mask to give the skin a rosy glow.

Zinc Oxide: This is a white, powdery mineral used in face powders, creams, and liquid foundations. Zinc oxide also has soothing properties and is used in ointments meant for burns, diaper rash, and insect bites. It is relatively nonallergenic.

Bibliography

Allen, Linda, ed. *The Look You Like.* A.M.A. Committee on Cutaneous Health and Cosmetics, 1966.

Angeloglou, Maggie. *The History of Make-up.* London: Macmillan, 1965.

Aronsohn, Richard, and Epstein, Richard. *The Miracle of Plastic Surgery.* Los Angeles: Shelbourne Press, 1970.

Blank, Irwin. "Action of Emollient Creams and Their Additives." *Journal of the American Medical Association,* CLXIV (May 25, 1957).

Bobroff, Arthur. *Acne.* Springfield, Ill.: Charles C. Thomas, 1964.

Burdick, H. "Chlorophyll in Cosmetics." *Journal of the Society of Cosmetic Chemists,* V (1954).

Donnan, Marcia. *Cosmetics from the Kitchen.* New York: Holt, Rinehart and Winston, 1972.

Dowling, Colette. *The Skin Game.* New York: Doubleday, 1971.

Eller, J. J., and Eller, W. D. "Estrogenic Ointments: Cutaneous Effects of Topical Applications of Natural Estrogens." *Archives of Dermatology and Syphilology,* LIX (1949).

Fisher, Alexander. *Contact Dermatitis.* Philadelphia: Lea and Febiger, 1967.

Flesch, Peter. "Chemistry of the Aging Skin." *Journal of the Society of Cosmetic Chemists,* VI (December 1955).

Foman, S. *Cosmetic Surgery: Principles and Practices.* Philadelphia: Lippincott, 1960.

Gohlke, Horst. "Use of Placenta Extracts in Cosmetics." *American Perfumer*, February 1954.

Goldsmidt, H. "Use of Milk in Cosmetics." *American Perfumer*, October 1946.

Greenberg, Leon, and Lester, David. *Handbook of Cosmetic Materials.* New York: Interscience, 1954.

Greenblatt, Robert, ed. *The Hirsute Female.* Springfield, Ill.: Charles C. Thomas, 1963.

Greenblatt, Robert, and Mahesh, Virendra. "Clinical Evaluation and Treatment of the Hirsute Female." *Clinical Obstetrics and Gynecology*, VII (December 1964).

Harry, Ralph G. *The Principles and Practices of Modern Cosmetics.* New York: Chemical Publishing, 1963.

Howard, Kenneth. "Uses of Enzymes in Cosmetics." *Journal of the Society of Cosmetic Chemists*, XIII (January 1962).

Howell, J. B. "Sunlight Factor in Aging and Skin Cancer." *Archives of Dermatology*, LXXXII (December 1960).

Humphrey, J., and White, R. *Immunology for Students of Medicine.* Philadelphia: F. A. Davis, 1963.

Ippen and Ippen. "Smoking, Aging and the Sun." *Journal of the Society of Cosmetic Chemists*, VI (May 1965).

Jacobi, O. "Nature of Cosmetic Films on the Skin." *Journal of the Society of Cosmetic Chemists*, XVIII (March 1967).

Janistyn, H. "Active Principle of Plants in Cosmetology." *American Perfumer*, January 1961.

Jellinek, Joseph S. *Formulation and Function of Cosmetics.* New York: Interscience, 1967.

Keithler, William. *The Formulation of Cosmetics and Cosmetic Specialties.* New York: Drug and Cosmetic Industry, 1956.

Klarmann, Emil. *Cosmetic Chemistry for Dermatologists.* Springfield, Ill.: Charles C. Thomas, 1962.

———. "Open Problem of Biological Activity in Cosmetics." *Journal of the Society of Cosmetic Chemists*, XVIII (February 1962).

Knox, John, Cockerell, E., and Freeman, R. "Etiological Factors and Premature Aging." *Journal of the American Medical Association*, CLXXIX (February 24, 1962).

Lerner, M., and Lerner, A. *Dermatologic Medications*. Chicago: Year Book Medical Publishers, 1960.

Linde, Shirley Motte, ed. *Cosmetic Surgery*. New York: Award Books, 1971.

Loriacz, Allan. "Physiological and Pathological Changes in Skin from Sunburn and Suntan." Presented at the symposium on sunlight and the skin at the Clinical Meeting of the A.M.A., Dallas, Texas, December 2, 1959. Reprinted by the A.M.A. Committee on Cutaneous Health and Cosmetics.

Lubowe, Irwin. "Modern Management of Hair and Scalp Disorders." *New York State Journal of Medicine*, June 1, 1966.

Lynfield, Y. "Effects of Pregnancy on the Human Hair Cycle." *Journal of Investigative Dermatology*, XXXV (December 1960).

Meyers, Earl. "New Drugs and the Cosmetic Chemist." *Journal of the Society of Cosmetic Chemists*, XVIII (December 1962).

Migeon, Claude. "Adrenal Androgens in Man." *The American Journal of Medicine*, LIII (November 1972).

Montagna, William, ed. *Advances in Biology of the Skin*, a series.
    Vol. 4 (with R. A. Ellis): *The Sebaceous Glands*. Oxford and New York: Pergamon Press, 1963.
    Vol. 5 (with Rupert E. Billingham): *Wound Healing*. Oxford and New York: Pergamon Press, 1964.
    Vol. 6: *Aging*. Oxford and New York: Pergamon Press, 1965.
    Vol. 9 (with Richard L. Dobson): *Hair Growth*. Oxford and New York: Pergamon Press, 1969.
    Vol. 10 (with Peter J. Bentley and Richard L. Dobson): *The Dermis*. New York: Appleton-Century-Crofts, 1970.

Morini, Simona. *Body Sculpture*. New York: Delacorte, 1972.

Navarre, Maison de. *The Chemistry and Manufacture of Cosmetics*. 2nd edn. Princeton, N.J.: Van Nostrand, 1962.

Papa, Christopher. "Effect of Topical Hormones on Aging Human Skin." *Journal of the Society of Cosmetic Chemists*, XVIII (August 19, 1967).

Pascher, Francis, ed. *Dermatologic Formulary*. New York: Hoeber Division of Harper and Row, 1957.

Peck, Samuel, and Klarmann, Emil. "Hormone Cosmetics." *Practitioner*, CLXXIII (August 1954).

Perloff, W., Channick, B., Suplick, B., and Carrington, E. "Clinical Management of Idiopathic Hirsutism (Adrenal Virilism)." *Journal of the American Medical Association,* CLXVII (August 1958).

Pillsbury, D., Shelley, W., and Kligman, A. *Cutaneous Medicine.* Philadelphia: W. B. Saunders, 1961.

Polunin, Ivan. "An Industrial Dermatosis Due to Enzyme Action." *Nature,* CLXVII (March 17, 1951).

Poucher, W. *Perfumes, Cosmetics and Soaps.* Princeton, N.J.: Van Nostrand, 1960.

Powitt, A. *Guide to Hair Structure and Chemistry.* New York: Milady, 1971.

Rapp, G. W. "Use of Chlorophyll Derivatives in the Cosmetics Industry." *Journal of the Society of Cosmetic Chemists,* IV (March 1953).

Rothman, Stephen, ed. *Physiology and Biochemistry of the Skin.* Chicago: University of Chicago Press, 1954.

Rubin, Saul. "Percutaneous Absorption of Vitamins." *Journal of the Society of Cosmetic Chemists,* XI (April 1960).

Sagarin, Edward, *et al. Cosmetics, Science and Technology.* New York: Interscience, 1957.

Savil, Agnes, and Warren, Clara. *The Hair and Scalp: A Clinical Study.* Baltimore: Williams and Wilkins, 1962.

Segre, Eugena. *Androgens, Virilization and the Hirsute Female.* Springfield, Ill.: Charles C. Thomas, 1967.

Smith, J. Graham, and Fenlagson, G. Rolland. "Dermal Connective Tissue Alterations with Age and Chronic Skin Damage." *Journal of the Society of Cosmetic Chemists,* XVI (August 1965).

Sperber, Perry. "Aging Skin and the Dermatologist." *Dermatological Digest,* May 1965.

————. *Treatment of the Aging Skin and Dermal Defects.* Springfield, Ill.: Charles C. Thomas, 1965.

Stabile, Toni. *Cosmetics: Trick or Treat?* New York: Hawthorn Books, 1966.

Sternberg, Thomas. *More Than Skin Deep.* New York: Doubleday, 1970.

Sternberg, Thomas, *et al. Evaluation of Therapeutic Agents and Cosmetics.* New York: McGraw-Hill, 1964.

Strauss, John, and Pochi, Peter. "Pathogenesis of Acne Vulgaris." *Journal of the Society of Cosmetic Chemists*, XIX (August 1968).

Sulzberger, M., Witten, V., and Kopf, A. "Diffuse Alopecia in Women: Its Unexplained Apparent Increase in Incidence." *Archives of Dermatology*, XVIII (April 1960).

Traven, Beatrice. *Here's Egg on Your Face.* Old Tappen, N.J.: Hewitt House, 1970.

Troy, William. "Changes in Human Skin in the Light of Current Theories of Aging." *Journal of the Society of Cosmetic Chemists*, XIX (December 9, 1968).

Urbach, Erich, and LeWinn, Edward. *Skin Diseases, Nutrition and Metabolism.* New York: Grune and Stratton, 1947.

Van Abbe, N., and Dean, Patricia. "Clinical Evaluation of Antidandruff Shampoos." *Journal of the Society of Cosmetic Chemists*, XVIII (July 1967).

Wells, F. V., and Lubowe, Irwin. *Cosmetics and the Skin.* New York: Van Nostrand, 1964.

Index

acid mantle, epidermis, 6–7; disturbance by cosmetics, cause of allergies, 120

acne, adolescent: care of skin, 55–60; causes, 51–5; cleansing of skin, 55–7; dermatologists' treatment techniques, 60–2; frequency, 51; grades of, 53–4; lotions or "medicated" foundations, 57; makeup, 58; outmoded treatments, 62–3; program of care for acned skin, 58–60; signs of, 51–4, and (Diagram 4) 52; toning of skin, 57–8; see also acne, postadolescent; acne scars

acne, postadolescent: drug-caused, 72–3; dry-skin, 71–2; hormonal, 73–6; mismanaged-skin, 68–70; see also acne, adolescent; acne scars; hormonal acne; mismanaged-skin acne

ACNE AID SOAP (Stiefel), 47, 69

ACNE-DOME (Dome), 57

acne lotions, function, 57

acne scars: (Diagram 5) 64; treatments for, description and evaluation, 64–7; types of, 63–4

ACNOMEL (Smith, Kline & French), 57

ACTH, acne caused by, 72

adrenal glands, 51; malfunction, cause of hirsutism, 142–3

aging skin: described, 88; drug use as cause, 137–8; smoking as cause, 134–5; sunlight as cause, 128–30; see also lined skin; wrinkles

air pollution, relation to oily skin, 46

ALBERTO VO 5 (Alberto-Culver), 196

ALBOLENE CREAM (Norcliff), 31, 113

alcohol: anti-acne soap ingredient, 56; value in skin care, 259

aldosterone, defined, 142

allantoin: definition and value in skin care, 259; treatment for red splotches in thin-skinned women, 112

allergic reactions: acute reactions, 114–15; delayed reactions, 116; drug users and, 137; eye-area problems caused by, 158–9, 160; persons susceptible to, 113; tests for reaction to hair-coloring products, 229–30; see also contact dermatitis; hypo-allergenic cosmetics

allergy: defined, 113–14; types, 114–16

allergy-tested cosmetics, hypo-allergenic value, 124

Almay: hypo-allergenic cosmetics, 122–3; labeling of products, 20; oil-free cosmetics, 48

ALMAY CREME RINSE (Almay), 192

almond oil: cause of contact dermatitis, 119; extract of oil of almond distinguished, 259; value in skin care, 259–60

alopecia areata, description of and treatment for, 209–10, 260; see also thin and thinning hair

althea, value in skin care, 260

alum, value in skin care, 21, 260

aluminum salts, cause of contact dermatitis, 118

aluminum sulfate, value in skin care, 260

Amerlate, natural moisturizing factor, 39

amino acids, value in skin care, 18, 260

AMINO-PON (Redken), 220, 226, 240

AMINO-PON K-11 (Redken), 257

ammonia, cause of contact dermatitis, 118

ammoniated mercury: cause of contact dermatitis, 118; value in skin care, 261

ammonium thioglycolate, permanent-waving solution, 244

amphetamines, use, effect on skin, 137

amyl nitrites, use, effect on skin, 137

androgens, definition and function, 51, 142

anemia: cause of dark circles under eyes, 161; sallow skin caused by, treatment for, 151–2

aniline dyes, value in hair care, 261; see also aniline hair dyes

aniline hair dyes: action on hair, 228–31, and (Diagram 27) 228; allergic reaction to, 118, 229–30; frosting with, 236–7; highlighting shampoo tints,

231–2; methods of using, 231–6; one-step tints, 233–4; shampoo-in tints, 232–3; streaking with, 236–7; tests for allergic reactions to, 229–30; two-step tints, 234–6; *see also* hair coloring; hair dyes

animal-embryo serum injections: fine lines, treatment for, 85; value in skin care, 267–8

animal fats, addition to skin creams, value, 16–17

anise, defined, 261

antihistamines, defined, 115, 117

antibodies, defined, 115

antiperspirants, contents and function, 25

antiseptic, defined, 261

apocrine glands, description and function, 9

apples, value in skin care, 261

apricot-kernel oil, value as skin-cream additive, 17

Aqualizer, natural moisturizing factor, 39

arcels, defined, 261

Ar-Ex cosmetics: hypo-allergenic, 122–3; oil-free, 48

arnica flowers, value in skin care, 261–2

artichoke, value in skin care, 262

aspirin rinse, dandruff treatment, 200

astringents: acned skin, choice for, 57, 59, 69; choice of, guide, 21; described, 20, 262; dry skin, homemade solutions for, recipes, 40–1, 44; fine lines, treatment for, 80–1; enlarged pores, effect on, (Diagram 20) 148; homemade, recipes, 40–1, 44, 49–50; ingredients, disclosure on label, 20–1; normal skin, choice for, 32; oily skin, choice for and recipe, 47, 49–50; rubefactant distinguished, 21; skin fresheners compared, 20; value in skin care, 262

attar of roses, defined, 262

Aveeno soap (Cooper), 116, 272

avocado, value in skin care, 262

Avon, labeling of products, 20

azulene, definition and value in skin care, 262

baby-fine hair, 215; aids for, 216–17; problems of, 215

baby oil, 112

baldness, *see* thin or thinning hair

balsam hair preparations: for naturally dry hair, 191; for "skinny" hair, 203; value of, 274

balm mint, 263

bananas, value in skin care, 263

barium salts, cause of contact dermatitis, 118

barrier level, epidermis, 5–6

Basis soap (Duke), 12, 31, 278

bath additives, description and evaluation, 24–5

bath oils, description and function, 24

bath powders, description and function, 25

bath salts, function and evaluation, 24

Beauvoir, Simone de, 90

beer, value in skin care, 271

beeswax, value in skin care, 263

betanapthanol, cause of contact dermatitis, 118

benzoic acid, value in skin care, 263

bergamot oil: cause of contact dermatitis, 119; value in skin care, 263

biostimulants, definition and value in skin care, 263–4

biotin, value in hair care, 264

birch, value in skin or hair care, 264

birth control pills, cause of acne, 72–3

blackhead, described, 52, and (Diagram 4A) 52; *see also* acne, adolescent

bleached hair, *see* hair coloring; processed hair

bleaching creams and lotions, freckle removal, 96

bleaching of facial or body hair, technique, 146–7

blood circulation, skin, 4–5, 7; increase in, red splotches caused by, description of and treatment for, 111–13; poor circulation, cause of sallow skin, 153

blood circulation, scalp, 166–7

blood vessels, broken, cause of little red lines, 97–8

bloodshot eyes, treatment for, 157–8

bluing rinse: for gray hair, recipe, 214; value in hair care, 264

body builders, hair, description and function, 180, 264

body hair: growth of, 140; shaving as removal method, 145; *see also* hirsutism

body lotions, 25

body wave, defined, 244; *see also* permanent-waving

borax, value in skin or hair care, 264

boric acid: cause of contact dermatitis, 118; definition and value, 264

bovine serum albumin, face coating based on, value, 81–2

Bravisol (Stiefel), 31, 47, 57

Breck Cream Rinse (Breck), 192, 195

Breck for Dry Hair (Breck), 197

Breck One (Breck), 241, 256

bromelin, defined, 22; *see also* keratolytic agents

brown spots, description, cause and removal methods, 95

Brush-On Peel-Off Mask (Helena Rubinstein), 81

brush-roller syndrome, treatment, 204–5

tion, 124–6; *see also names of specific types of cosmetics*

cottonseed oil, sunscreen ingredient, 131

cream conditioners, hair, description and function, 180–1

creaming of face, factor in wrinkled skin, 89

cream rinses, hair: description and function, 179; dyed hair, danger to, 242–3; naturally dry hair, 191–2

cresylic compounds, cause of contact dermatitis, 119

cucumber, value in skin care, 267

cuticle, hair-strand layer, described, 165, and (Diagram 25) 170; factor in shine of hair, 170–1; roughing up, baby-fine hair, 216–17

cyst, described, 53, and (Diagram 4D) 52; *see also* acne, adolescent

dandruff: described, 198; dry-scalp, description of and treatment for, 199–200; dyed hair, treatment for, 241; gray or graying hair, 197–8; normal-scalp, treatment for, 200; oily-scalp, causes of and treatment for, 198–9; straightened hair, shampoo for, 257; tension as cause, 200–1; *see also* shampoos

Daniell, Dr. Harry W., 134–5

day creams: additives, value of, 39; description and evaluation, 16; dry skin, choice for, 38–40; oil additives, value of, 16–17

daytime lotions, description and evaluation, 16

Deep Mist Gentle Gel Mask (Almay), 33

Deep Mist Toning and Refining Lotion (Almay), 32

deodorants, contents and function, 25

deodorant soaps, description and evaluation, 12

depilatories, description and function, 145

dermabrasion: acne or acne scars, treatment for, 64; brown spots, removal by, 95; fine lines, treatment for, 87; freckles, removal by, 96

dermatologist-tested cosmetics, hypo-allergenic value, 124

dermis: blood vessels, 4–5, 7; collagen fibers, *see* collagen; described, 7, and (Diagram 3) 7; oil glands, description and function, 8–9; *see also* epidermis; skin (generally)

developers, hair-dye solution, defined, 267

diet: acne, relation to, 54; iron-rich foods, list, 152–3; low-sodium diet, 74–5; oily skin, relation to, 45–6; protein-rich foods essential to hair

growth, list, 208–9

dilantin, acne caused by, 72–3

doctor-approved cosmetics, hypo-allergenic value, 124

doctor-tested cosmetics, hypo-allergenic value, 124

Domeboro Powder (Dome), 112

Dove Soap (Lever Brothers), 12, 31, 112, 272

drabber, defined, 232

drinking, excessive: effect on skin, 136; little red lines, cause of, 97; skin-care program for drinkers, 136; wrinkling of skin, factor in, 88

drug-caused acne, description, 72–3

drug use, habitual, effect on skin, 137–8

dry hair: after processing, description and care, 192–4; curly, coarse, "dry" hair, description and care, 194–6; gray or graying hair, care of, 196–8; hard-water rinse for, recipe, 223–4; naturally dry hair, description, causes and care, 190–2

dry-scalp drandruff, description of and treatment for, 191, 199–200

dry skin: acid mantle, disturbance, cause of allergies to cosmetics, 120; acned skin, 71–2; after age 30, profile of, 28; althea infusion for, recipe, 260; astringent for, homemade, recipe, 40–1; care of, 37–44; cause of, 5; 35–6; day creams, choice for, 38–40; drinker's skin, care program, 136–7; enlarged pores, treatment for, 148–9; face masks for, 41; facial saunas for, 41; makeup for, 41–2; management, considerations in, 36–7; oil-balance control, 38–40; popular emphasis on, 35; program of care for, 42–3; red splotches in thin-skinned women, treatment for, 112; smoker's skin, care program, 135; toning of, 40–2; youthful, profile of, 27–8

dry-skin acne: description and profile, 71–2; treatment for, 72

dull hair: hard water as cause, homemade care preparations, recipes, 223–4; melanin content as cause, 214; oiliness as cause, 222; processing as cause, 222

dyed hair: cream rinses, dangers of, 252–3; dandruff treatment for, 241; herb-based products, use on, effect, 243; permanent-waving, "crash" care program prior to, 242; sun damage, protection from, 241; *see also* hair coloring; hair dyes; processed hair

eccrine glands, description and function, 9

eggs: value in skin care, 19, 267; shampoos, 178

egg whites, face masks using, treatment for fine lines, 81

elder, value in skin care, 267

electric needles: brown spots, removal by, 95; fine lines, treatment for, 84–5

electrical stimulation, effect on lined skin, 83

electrolysis, described, 145

embryo serum, *see* animal-embryo serum injections

ENDEN (Helene Curtis), 197

environment, relation to oily skin, 46

epidermis: acid mantle, 6–7; barrier level, 5–6; basal layer, 4–5; blood supply to, 4–5; described, 3–7, and (Diagram 1) 3; layers of, 4–7; upper layer, 6; *see also* dermis; skin (generally)

essential oils, cause of contact dermatitis, 119

estrogen: secretion of, 51; value in skin care, 23, 268; *see also* estrogen creams; hormone therapy

estrogen creams: availability, 39; fine lines, treatment for, 80; facial hair growth as caused by, 144–5; *see also* hormone therapy

ethnic background: hirsutism, factor in, 144; oily skin, factor in, 46; thin skin, factor in, 111; wrinkled skin, factor in, 88

Everything You Want to Know About Salt-free Recipes (Nancy Lloyd), 75

exfoliating lotions, *see* clarifying lotions

exhaustion, cause of sallow skin, 153

EXTRA RICH FACIAL PACK (Shiseido), 41, 81

EXTREME PROTEIN PACK (Redken), 251, 257

eye area: circles under eyes, causes of and treatment for, 160–1; lined and baggy tissue, causes of and treatment for, 159–60; puffy lids, causes of and treatment for, 158–9; undereye bags, removal by face-lift operation, 92, and (Diagram 7) 92; upper eyelid, tightening by facelift operation, 92, and (Diagram 7) 92

eyebrow dyes, cautions, 229, 231

eye creams, value of, 40, 268

eyelash dyes: cautions, 229, 231; false lashes, wearing after face lift, 94

eyes: bloodshot, treatment for, 157–8; excessive tearing, treatment for, 158

face-lift operation: aging skin, treatment by, 90–1; basic technique described, 91–3, and (Diagrams 6–8) 91–3; postoperative care, 93–4; repetition, frequency of, 94; results of, 93–4, and (Diagram 8) 93; skin care following healing, 93–4; undereye bags, removal, 92, and (Diagram 7) 92; upper eyelid, tightening of, 92, and (Diagram 7) 92; *see also* cosmetic surgery

face masks: acned skin, choice for, 58, 59, 69; additives, value of, 23; dry skin, choice for, 41, 44; fine lines, treatment for, 81; homemade, recipes, 34, 44; normal skin, choice for, 32–3, 34; oily skin, choice for, 47–8; types of, 22–3; value in skin toning, 22–3; *see also* toning of skin

face massage: after face lift, 94; lined skin, effect on, 83; wrinkled skin, factor in, 89

facial angles: "ideal" angles, 99–102, and (Diagram 10) 101; too large angle between forehead and nose, correction by surgery, 107, and (Diagram 17) 107; *see also* facial features

facial cephalogram, defined, 102

facial expressions, factor in wrinkled skin, 89

facial features: alteration by cosmetic surgery, moral discussion, 108–10; angles formed by, *see* facial angles; proportions, "ideal," 99–102, and (Diagram 9) 100; *see also names of specific features of face*

facial hair: excess hair, what constitutes, 139–40; growth of, described, 140; removal of excess, methods, 145–6; *see also* hirsutism

facial muscles, relation to lined skin, 79, 83

FACIAL PACK (Shiseido), 33

FACIAL PACK (EXTRA RICH) (Shiseido), 41, 81

facial saunas: acned skin, 69; additives, necessity for, 23; description and function, 23; dry-skin care, 41; fine lines, treatment for, 81; homemade, described, 23; normal skin, use for, 33; oily skin, use for, 48; value of, 23–4

fat pads, face, effect of loss of, 88

fatty acids, value in skin or hair care, 268

fennel, value in skin care, 268

fenugreek, value in skin care, 268

Filatov extracts, *see* biostimulants

filler, hair dye, defined, 268

fine lines: animal-embryo serum injections, treatment with, 85; astringents for, 80; care of, 78, 79–83; causes, 77–8; chemical-peeling as treatment, 85–7; cosmetic care, 78, 79–83; dermabrasion as treatment, 87; electric needles, treatment with, value, 84–5; face masks for, 81; sun damage as cause, 78–9; wear and tear on skin as cause, 78–9; *see also* lined skin; wrinkles

5-MINUTE COLOR (Clairol), 232

5-MINUTE FACIAL MASK (Almay), 58

formaldehyde, cause of contact dermatitis, 119
FOSTEX soap (Westwood), 56
FOSTRIL (Westwood), 47, 57
freckles: defined, 95–6; removal, methods, 96
French milled soaps, description and evaluation, 12
freshening lotions, *see* skin fresheners
frosting of hair, described, 236–7
fruits, addition to soaps, effect, 13

galvanic current, value as acne treatment, 66
gel-type face masks: described, 22–3; dry skin, choice for, 41; fine lines, treatment for, 81; normal skin, choice for, 32–3; *see also* face masks
genetics: acne, relation to, 55; oily skin, relation to, 46
ginger, wild, value in beauty care, 279
ginseng, value in skin care, 268
glue sniffing, effect on skin, 137
glutamic acid, value in skin care, 269; *see also* amino acids
glycerin, value in skin care, 269
grapefruit, value in skin care, 269
grapes, value in skin care, 269
gray and graying hair: bluing rinse for, recipe, 214; care programs for, 197, 214–15; coloring, 213, 225, 232, 236, 237; dandruff, treatment for, 197–8; description, 212; drying and coarsening, 214; dullness, in fair-haired women, 224; frosting of, 236–7; hot-oil treatment for, 197; premature graying, causes, 212; processed hair, care of, 198; streaking of, 236–7; vitamin B therapy, value, 212; yellowish tinge, causes and removal, 214
green soap, value in skin care, 269

hair body builders, description and function, 180, 264
hairbrushes and combs: condition of, for avoidance of split ends, 221; washing of, 174–5
hair brushing and combing, techniques, 174–5
hair bulb, scalp, 167
hair care: baby-fine hair, 216–17; basics, 174–86; brushing and combing, techniques, 174–5; *see also* hair-care programs; hair conditioners; hair conditioning; hair setting; scalp massage; shampooing; shampoos
hair-care programs: for bleached hair, 240; for curly, coarse, "dry" hair, 195–6; for gray hair, dry and coarse, 214–15; for naturally dry hair, 192; for permanented hair, 249–51; for split ends, 220–1; for straightened hair, 257; *see*

also hair care
hair color: change in, 173; factors determining, 172–3; *see also* hair coloring
hair coloring: after face lift, 94; allergic reactions, tests for, 229–30; baby-fine hair, remedy for, 216–17; do's and don't's, list, 230–1; gray hair, 213, 225, 232, 236, 237; permanent color, 226; processed hair, problems with, 237–8; semi-permanent color, 226; "skinny" hair, remedy for, 202–3; sunburst effect, 237; sun-damaged hair, 219–20; temporary color, 225–6; *see also* aniline hair dyes; dyed hair; hair dyes; processed hair
hair conditioners: dry, processed hair, 194; naturally dry hair, 191–2; oily hair, 189; types and functions, 179–81; *see also* hair conditioning
hair conditioning: hot-oil treatment, described, 250–1; permanented hair, 249–51; sun-damaged hair, reconditioning, 219; *see also* hair care; hair-care programs; hair conditioners
hair dyes, 226–31; certified color, defined, 225, 266; developers, defined, 267; filler, defined, 268; metallic dyes, described, 227–8; removal procedure, metallic and vegetable dyes, 227–8; vegetable dyes, described, 227; *see also* aniline hair dyes; dyed hair; hair coloring
hair elasticity: factors determining, 172; permanent-waving, consideration in, 172
hair follicle: curly hair, 168, and (Diagram 24E) 169; straight hair, 168, and (Diagram 24D) 169; *see also* hair growth
hair growth: formation in scalp, 166–7, and (Diagram 22) 166; growth cycle, 166–7, and (Diagram 23) 167; protein-rich foods essential to, list, 208–9; *see also* facial hair
hair length: factors determining, 171; hair straightening, factor in, 255; permanent-waving, factor in, 246–7
hair loss, *see* thin and thinning hair
hair porosity: hair straightening, factor in, 254; permanent-waving, factor in, 245–6
hair problems: baby-fine hair, 215–17; dull hair, causes of and treatment for, 222–4; "skinny" hair, causes of and treatment for, 202–3; split ends, causes of and treatment for, 220–1; *see also* dandruff; thin and thinning hair
hair setting: basic procedure, 184; curly, coarse, "dry" hair, 196; electric rollers, use of, 184–5; hair-shaft structure, effect on, 183; rules for, 183–4; split ends, prevention of, 221

hair shaft: composition of. 165–6, and (Diagram 21) 166; curly or kinky hair, 168–70, and (Diagram 24C&E) 169; protein molecules, arrangement, 182, and (Diagram 26) 182; straight hair, 168–70, and (Diagram 24A&D) 169; thickness, factor in hair processing, 246, 255; wavy hair, 168–70, and (Diagram 24B) 169

hair shine: factors determining, 170; *see also* dull hair

hair straightening: avoidance, method of, 195–6; care of straightened hair, 256–7; hennaed hair, 227; home vs. salon, 256; precautions, 256; procedure, 252–4; success of, determining factors, 254–5; sun-damaged hair, 219–20; *see also* processed hair

hair type: curly or kinky, 168–70, and (Diagram 24C&E) 169; straight, 168–70, and (Diagram 24A&D) 169; wavy, 168–70, and (Diagram 24B) 169

hair volume: factors determining, 171–2; hair straightening, factor in, 255; increase in, methods of, 172; permanent-waving, factor in, 246; *see also* thin and thinning hair

hand creams, contents, 269

HAPPY FACE (Tussy), 31

hard-water areas, preparations for use in: homemade hair preparations, recipes, 223–4; soaps, composition, 269–70

hazelnut, value in skin care, 270

HEAD & SHOULDERS (Lever Brothers), 199, 241

heat, exposure to, cause of little red lines, 97

Helena Rubinstein, hair-color highlighting products, 226

hemaglobin, function in skin color, 151

henna, 227, 270; removal procedure, 227–8; *see also* hair coloring

herb-based preparations: cosmetics, hypo-allergenic value, 124; dyed hair, discoloration by, 243; hair rinses, description, function, and recipe, 179–80; face masks, value, 23; shampoos, value, 178; soaps, value, 13

heredity, *see* genetics

heroin, habitual use, effect on skin, 137

high blood pressure, cause of little red lines, 97

hirsutism: cortisone therapy for, 144; ethnic background as factor, 144; genetics as factor, 144; hormone imbalance as cause, 140–3; other causes, 143–5; ovaries, malfunction of as cause, 140–2; postmenopausal, 144; treatments and hair-removal methods, 144–7; *see also* facial hair

histamines, defined, 115

honey-based products: value in skin care, 270; face masks, 23, 81; night creams, 19

hops, value in skin care, 271

hormo-fruit extracts, defined, 270

hormonal acne: kinds of, 72; medical problem causing, symptoms of and treatment for, 75–6; nonspecific imbalance causing, profile of and treatment for, 73–5; *see also* acne, post-adolescent

hormone balance: effect on skin, 36–7; oily skin, relation to, 45; *see also* hormone imbalance

hormone creams, availability, 39; *see also* estrogen creams; hormone therapy

hormone imbalance: allergies to cosmetics, cause of, 120; hirsutism, cause of, 140; Male-pattern Baldness (MPB), cause of, 210–11; *see also* hormone balance

hormones, production of, relation to acne, 51–2, 142–3; *see also names of specific hormones; e.g.,* cortisone, estrogen

hormone therapy: acne, treatment for, 73–5; dry-skin care, value in, 37; water retention due to. low-sodium diet, 74–5

horsetail, value in skin or hair care, 270

hot-oil treatment, hair, 250–1

hot packs, anti-acne treatment, 56

hot weather, relation to acne, 55

hydrogen bonds, in hair shaft, definition and function, 182

hydrogen peroxide, value in skin or hair care, 270

hyperkeratinization, defined, 198; *see also* dandruff

hypo-allergenic cosmetics: Almay products, ingredients omitted, list, 123; Ar-Ex products, 122–3; definition, 122; persons requiring, 126–7; *see also* allergic reactions

"ice pick" scars, 63, and (Diagram 5A) 63; *see also* acne scars

INH, acne caused by, 72–3

INNOCENT COLOR (Toni), 232

Irish moss, value in skin care, 265

iron-rich foods, list, 152–3

juniper, value in skin care, 270

keratin, defined, 5

keratinization, defined, 5

keratolytic agents: defined, 22; labels, disclosure on, 22

labeling of products, disclosure of in-

A Note About the Author

In 1963, Deborah Chase was chosen as one of the seven top young scientists in the country by the Westinghouse Science Talent Search—after winning twenty-five prizes for original scientific research as a student at the Bronx High School of Science. At New York University she was trained in biology and basic medical science and science writing. She has done research on aging, at New York University Medical Center, and on viruses, under grants from the National Institutes of Health. She and her husband, Dr. Neil Schachter, chief of Inhalation Therapy at Yale–New Haven Hospital, live with their two-year-old daughter, Karen Elizabeth, in New Haven.

A Note on the Type

The text of this book was set on the Linotype in Aster, a type face designed by Francesco Simoncini (born 1912 in Bologna, Italy) for Ludwig and Mayer, the German type foundry. Starting out with the basic old-face letterforms that can be traced back to Francesco Griffo in 1495, Simoncini emphasized the diagonal stress by the simple device of extending diagonals to the full height of the letterforms and squaring off. By modifying the weights of the individual letters to combat this stress, he has produced a type of rare balance and vigor. Introduced in 1958, Aster has steadily grown in popularity wherever type is used.